PEPTIDE PRESCRIPTION

AN INTRODUCTION TO PEPTIDE THERAPY, A CLINICIAN'S RESOURCE

DR. SOLOMON JAN

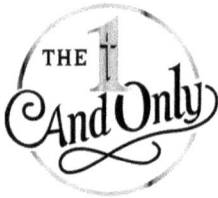

To my parents—
You were God's greatest gift to my journey,
guiding me with prayer, love, and quiet strength.
May this work reflect the light you placed in me.
Thanking you will never be enough.

CONTENTS

Appendices: References & Glossary

INTRODUCTION
WHY I WROTE THIS BOOK

I'VE SPENT OVER TWENTY YEARS IN MEDICINE—FIRST IN FAMILY practice, now in integrative and aesthetic care. Along the way, I've witnessed both the incredible power and the profound limitations of traditional medicine. People don't just want to survive; they want to thrive. They want to feel strong, youthful, vibrant, and fully alive—and that's where peptides and whole-person health come in.

This book exists because I'm tired of watching qualified medical professionals get overshadowed by YouTube personalities and self-proclaimed "experts" who lack the clinical training and real-world experience to guide people safely through their health optimization journey. Don't get me wrong—I respect anyone genuinely trying to help people improve their lives. But when it comes to your health, you deserve guidance from someone who has spent decades studying the human body, who understands the intricate dance of biochemistry, and who takes full responsibility for real patient outcomes.

I'm Dr. Solomon Jan. I'm board-certified in family medicine and serve as an Associate Professor of Medicine at the Medical University of South Carolina Florence and Marion, where I teach medical students and physician assistant students. I've treated thousands of patients at Grand Strand Medical Center and MUSC Health Marion Medical Center. I founded the International Society of Aesthetic and Regenerative Medicine, and I'm the President of sjan ventures, a consulting and coaching firm. More importantly, I've spent the last several years pioneering the clinical application of peptide therapy in my practice at Viva La Skin in Myrtle Beach, South Carolina.

But here's what really drives me, what keeps me awake at night and gets me up early in the morning: I was trained to diagnose and treat, but after years in practice, I realized I wasn't helping people heal. I was managing symptoms, prescribing medications, following protocols that were designed to keep people stable rather than help them flourish. My patients weren't thriving—they were surviving, and many were barely doing that.

The current healthcare system is fundamentally broken. We wait for people to get sick, then we treat the sickness. We focus on disease management rather than health optimization. We see patients as collections of symptoms rather than complex human beings with unique histories, genetics, environments, and needs. We've become so specialized that we've lost sight of the forest for the trees.

Meanwhile, people are suffering. They're dealing with chronic fatigue that no amount of sleep seems to fix. They're struggling with brain fog that makes them feel like shadows of their former selves. They're gaining weight despite eating less and exercising more. They're aging rapidly, watching their vitality slip away year by year, and being told this is "normal."

It's not normal. It's not acceptable. And it's not inevitable.

That frustration led me to look beyond the traditional playbook. It led me to study hormone optimization, nutrient therapy, and eventually, the emerging science of peptide therapy. Peptides—short chains of amino acids that act as cellular messengers—represent one of the most exciting frontiers in regenerative medicine. These tiny but mighty compounds help your body repair, regenerate, and optimize itself from the inside out.

But peptides aren't magic bullets. They're sophisticated tools that work best when integrated into a comprehensive approach that considers your genetics, your emotional health, your environment, your past traumas, your lifestyle patterns, and your unique biochemical needs. True healing requires us to see you as a whole human being, not just a diagnosis or a set of lab values.

This book is here to educate, to inspire, and to help you take the next step in your own health journey. Whether you're dealing with stubborn weight gain, chronic fatigue, hormonal imbalances, cognitive decline, or you simply want to age more gracefully and live your most optimal life, the science and stories in these pages will show you what's possible when we move beyond the limitations of conventional medicine.

You deserve to feel your best. You deserve to work with practitioners who see you as a whole human being worthy of comprehensive care. You deserve to know about cutting-edge tools like peptide therapy that can help you achieve levels of health and vitality you may have thought were impossible. And you deserve accurate, science-based information from practitioners who understand the complexities of the human body and take responsibility for patient safety.

The field of peptide therapy and integrative health is exploding with information—some good, much of it misleading or potentially dangerous. I see people without medical training positioning themselves as experts in complex biochemical interventions. I see patients trying to navigate this field without proper guidance, sometimes putting their health at risk by purchasing unregulated compounds online or following protocols designed by people who've never treated a patient.

That ends now. This book will give you the knowledge you need to be an informed advocate for your own health. You'll learn what questions to ask potential providers, how to evaluate treatment options, and how to build a comprehensive approach to health optimization that goes far beyond any single intervention.

This isn't about quick fixes or miracle cures. It's about understanding your body, optimizing your health, and working with qualified practitioners who have the training, experience, and commitment to help you achieve your goals safely and effectively.

The future of medicine is personalized, preventative, and regenerative. It addresses root causes instead of just managing symptoms. It recognizes that true health encompasses physical, emotional, and spiritual well-being. It empowers patients to be active participants in their own healing rather than passive recipients of treatments.

That future is available now, for those who are ready to embrace it. The question isn't whether you deserve to feel your best—you absolutely do. The question is: are you ready to take the next step toward your optimal health?

CHAPTER 1
THE AWAKENING OF A HEALER

"There has to be more than this."

T HAT THOUGHT HAUNTED ME FOR YEARS DURING MY TIME AS A family medicine physician. It would hit me at random moments— while writing yet another prescription for a medication that would mask symptoms without addressing root causes, while explaining to a patient that their debilitating fatigue was "probably just stress," while watching someone I genuinely wanted to help leave my office with the same problems they came in with.

I was doing everything right according to my medical training. I had graduated from medical school, completed my residency, passed my boards, and was practicing evidence-based medicine. I was follow-ing protocols, ordering appropriate labs, prescribing treatments that were backed by clinical studies. By every conventional measure, I was a successful physician.

But deep down, I knew I wasn't really helping people heal. I was managing their symptoms, keeping them stable, helping them survive—but they weren't thriving. And increasingly, I could see that they knew it too.

THE DAILY REALITY OF TRADITIONAL MEDICINE

Let me paint you a picture of what a typical day looked like during my years in traditional family medicine. The schedule was packed— fifteen-minute appointment slots with barely enough time to address the chief complaint, let alone explore the complex web of factors that might be contributing to a patient's health issues.

A forty-five-year-old executive would come in complaining of crushing fatigue, brain fog, and unexplained weight gain around his midsection. He'd tell me he used to feel sharp and energetic, but now he could barely make it through the day without multiple cups of coffee. He was gaining weight despite eating less and trying to exercise more. His sleep was fragmented, his mood was low, and his wife was starting to worry about him.

I'd order the standard battery of tests: complete blood count, comprehensive metabolic panel, thyroid function, maybe a testosterone level if I had time to think about it. His labs would come back "normal"—testosterone on the lower end of the range but technically within reference limits, thyroid function adequate, basic metabolic panel unremarkable. According to traditional medicine, there was nothing wrong with him.

My options were limited and frankly unsatisfying. I could suggest lifestyle modifications—get more sleep (easier said than done), try to exercise more (despite his fatigue), maybe eat a Mediterranean diet. If he seemed particularly down, I might consider an antidepressant. If his testosterone was really low, I might refer him to an endocrinologist who would likely tell him he didn't meet the criteria for replacement therapy.

But I could see in his eyes that he wasn't just looking for lifestyle advice. He was looking for answers. He was looking for someone to help him understand why a previously healthy, active person was suddenly feeling like a shadow of his former self. He was looking for someone to help him feel like himself again.

The same frustrating pattern repeated itself daily with remarkable consistency. Women struggling with hormonal chaos after childbirth or during perimenopause, being told their symptoms were "normal" or "part of getting older." Young adults with digestive issues that didn't fit neatly into diagnostic categories, bouncing from specialist to specialist without getting relief. Elderly patients whose "normal aging" seemed to accelerate despite our best efforts, losing muscle mass, cognitive function, and independence at rates that seemed neither normal nor acceptable.

THE MOMENT I REALIZED SOMETHING WAS FUNDAMENTALLY WRONG

The breaking point came with a patient I'll never forget—a fifty-two-year-old teacher named Margaret. She had been coming to see me for three years with complaints of fatigue, weight gain, joint pain, and what she described as "feeling like I'm disappearing." Her labs were consistently normal. Her physical exams were unremarkable. According to traditional medicine, she was fine.

But Margaret wasn't fine. She was struggling to get through her school days, falling asleep on the couch every evening, gaining weight despite carefully controlling her diet, and feeling like her body was betraying her. She had seen multiple specialists—rheumatologists, endocrinologists, psychiatrists—and everyone told her the same thing: her tests were normal, so there wasn't really anything wrong.

During one particular visit, Margaret broke down in tears.

"Doctor," she said, "I know something is wrong with me. I know my body better than any test, and I know this isn't normal. I feel like I'm dying from the inside out, but everyone keeps telling me I'm fine. Am I going crazy?"

In that moment, I realized that our entire system was failing this woman. We had reduced her to a series of numbers on lab reports, and because those numbers fell within predetermined ranges, we had decided she was healthy. But she wasn't healthy—she was suffering, and our narrow focus on pathology was preventing us from seeing the full picture of her human experience.

That's when I started to understand that traditional medicine, for all its strengths, was fundamentally reactive. We waited for people to get sick enough for their lab values to fall outside normal ranges, and then we treated the abnormal lab values. But what about the vast territory between optimal health and diagnosable disease? What about helping people thrive, not just survive?

THE FIRST STEPS BEYOND CONVENTIONAL MEDICINE

My journey beyond traditional medicine began during a particularly challenging period in my career. A group of physician colleagues and I had been discussing the possibility of starting a side business—something that would allow us to escape the constraints and frustrations of traditional medicine while still using our medical training to help people.

But it was a devastating personal experience that truly catalyzed my transition. Just sixteen months out of my fellowship training, while serving as director of a nursing home, I was hit with my first lawsuit. The case involved a patient I had cared for, and despite doing everything according to standard protocols, I found myself in the crosshairs of the legal system. That moment shook me to my core and made me realize how vulnerable physicians are in the traditional healthcare system, no matter how carefully and conscientiously we practice.

In that moment of uncertainty and frustration, aesthetics seemed like a potential lifeline—a way for me to leave traditional medicine behind, support my family, and actually have fun practicing medicine again. It represented freedom from the bureaucratic constraints, legal vulnerabilities, and systemic limitations that were making traditional practice increasingly difficult.

As I began studying aesthetic procedures and spending time with patients who were seeking cosmetic treatments, I discovered something that fundamentally changed my perspective. The patients who had the best outcomes from aesthetic procedures weren't just receiving isolated cosmetic treatments—they were optimizing their health from the inside out.

These patients understood that true beauty and vitality came from comprehensive wellness. They were working with providers who looked at hormone levels, nutritional status, sleep quality, stress management, and overall health optimization as integral parts of achieving their aesthetic goals. They were investing in themselves holistically, and the results were remarkable—not just in how they looked, but in how they felt.

This realization led me to dive deeper into hormone replacement therapy. I started learning about the intricate ways that hormones influence not just reproductive function, but energy levels, cognitive performance, body composition, mood, sleep quality, and overall vitality. I began to understand how hormonal imbalances could explain many of the "normal" symptoms I had been dismissing in my family medicine practice.

But it was my discovery of peptide therapy that truly revolutionized my understanding of what was possible in medicine.

DISCOVERING THE POWER OF PEPTIDES

My introduction to peptides came through an unexpected conversation with a colleague in the emergency department. He had been scheduled for back surgery—a procedure that would have meant months of recovery and uncertainty about whether he'd be able to return to his demanding work in the ER. But instead of going under the knife, he had stumbled upon peptides while researching alternative treatment options.

"Solomon," he told me, "I was desperate to avoid surgery, so I started looking into everything—acupuncture, physical therapy, you name it. Then I came across these things called peptides. I figured I had nothing to lose, so I tried them. Six months later, my back pain is completely gone. I avoided surgery altogether."

This piqued my interest immediately. Here was a fellow physician—someone trained in evidence-based medicine—telling me about compounds that had literally changed the trajectory of his health and career. I had to know more.

I started researching peptides extensively, diving into the scientific literature and learning about these short chains of amino acids that act as signaling molecules in the body. But more than just studying them, I decided to try them myself. If I was going to recommend these compounds to patients, I needed to understand firsthand how they worked and what effects they might have.

I started with basic tissue repair and recovery peptides, monitoring my own response carefully. The results were subtle at first, but over time I noticed improvements in my energy levels, recovery from workouts, and overall sense of well-being. This personal experience convinced me that there was something significant here worth exploring further.

From there, I expanded my knowledge base, studying different types of peptides, their mechanisms of action, safety profiles, and clinical applications. The more I learned, the more excited I became about their potential. Here were compounds that could stimulate natural growth hormone production, enhance tissue repair, improve cognitive function, support weight management, boost immune function, and promote longevity—all by working with the body's existing systems rather than against them.

But what really convinced me to integrate peptides into my practice were the results I started seeing with my own patients.

THE TRANSFORMATION THAT CHANGED EVERYTHING

One of my early peptide therapy patients was a woman named Sarah, a fifty-four-year-old marketing executive who had been struggling with weight gain, insulin resistance, and crushing fatigue for several years. She had seen multiple doctors, tried every diet imaginable, and even worked with a personal trainer, but nothing seemed to help. Traditional medicine had offered her metformin for her pre-diabetes, a recommendation to "eat less and exercise more," and the general sense that this was just part of getting older.

When Sarah first came to see me, she was desperate. "Dr. Jan," she said, "I feel like I'm disappearing. I used to be energetic, confident, and strong. Now I can barely make it through the day without a nap, I've gained forty pounds that won't come off no matter what I do, and I feel like my brain is wrapped in cotton. Everyone tells me this is normal for my age, but it doesn't feel normal to me."

I performed a comprehensive assessment that went far beyond traditional lab work. We looked at her hormone levels, inflammatory markers, nutrient status, sleep quality, stress patterns, and metabolic function. We also explored her history—past traumas, life stressors, environmental exposures, and emotional health.

What we discovered was a complex picture of hormonal imbalance, insulin resistance, chronic inflammation, and a nervous system stuck in fight-or-flight mode due to years of chronic stress. Her cortisol patterns were completely dysregulated, her growth hormone production had plummeted, and her cellular repair mechanisms were significantly impaired.

Based on this comprehensive assessment, I designed a personalized protocol that included specific peptides targeted at her individual needs. We used GLP-1 receptor agonists to help with weight management and insulin sensitivity, growth hormone-releasing peptides to support her natural hormone production, and anti-inflammatory peptides to help her body heal from years of chronic stress.

But the peptides were just one part of a comprehensive approach. We also optimized her other hormones, addressed her nutritional deficiencies, implemented stress management techniques, and worked on healing the emotional and psychological factors that were contributing to her health issues.

The transformation was remarkable. Within six weeks, Sarah's energy levels began to improve. By three months, she had lost twenty-five pounds and her brain fog had completely cleared. Her sleep improved dramatically, her mood stabilized, and her lab values showed a complete reversal of her insulin resistance and inflammatory markers.

But more importantly than any single metric, Sarah felt like herself again. She had reclaimed her energy, her confidence, and her sense of vitality. She didn't just lose weight—she reclaimed her life.

UNDERSTANDING THE HOLISTIC PICTURE

Sarah's transformation taught me something crucial: peptides work best when they're part of a comprehensive, holistic approach to health. It's not enough to simply prescribe a compound and hope for the best. True healing requires us to understand and address the complex web of factors that influence health and disease.

I started to recognize patterns in my patients that traditional medicine had taught me to ignore or dismiss. The successful business-woman whose chronic inflammation and autoimmune symptoms didn't improve despite perfect lab values until we addressed her history of childhood trauma. The athlete whose performance plateaued until we discovered and treated a chronic gut infection that was triggering systemic inflammation. The menopausal woman whose hot flashes and mood swings resolved not just with hormone replacement, but with peptides that helped her body produce and utilize hormones more effectively.

Each patient taught me something new about the intricate connections between physical health, emotional well-being, environmental factors, genetic predispositions, and life experiences. I began to understand that true healing requires us to see each person as a unique individual with a complex history and specific needs, rather than as a diagnosis or a set of symptoms to be managed.

This is what twenty years in medicine taught me: the human body is incredibly sophisticated, and true healing requires us to respect that sophistication. We can't just treat symptoms—we have to understand the underlying causes. We can't just focus on one system—we have to consider how all the systems interact. We can't just address the physical—we have to acknowledge the emotional, mental, and spiritual aspects of health.

THE SCIENCE BEHIND THE SUCCESS

As I witnessed more and more transformations in my practice, I became increasingly passionate about understanding the science behind these remarkable results. Peptides work through multiple mechanisms that support the body's natural healing and optimization processes.

Growth hormone-releasing peptides, for example, stimulate the pituitary gland to produce more growth hormone naturally, which supports muscle growth, fat loss, tissue repair, and overall vitality. Unlike synthetic growth hormone, which can shut down natural production, these peptides enhance the body's own hormone production systems.

GLP-1 receptor agonists work by mimicking hormones that regulate blood sugar and appetite, helping people achieve sustainable weight loss while improving metabolic health. But they also have effects on the brain, reducing inflammation and potentially supporting cognitive function.

Tissue repair peptides like BPC-157 have been shown to accelerate healing of everything from muscle and tendon injuries to gastrointestinal damage. They work by enhancing the body's natural repair mechanisms rather than simply masking pain or inflammation.

Cognitive enhancement peptides can cross the blood-brain barrier and support neurotransmitter function, helping people achieve better focus, memory, and mental clarity. They're particularly valuable for people dealing with brain fog, age-related cognitive decline, or the mental effects of chronic stress.

The beauty of peptide therapy is that these compounds work synergistically with the body's existing systems. Instead of forcing artificial changes, they support and enhance natural processes. This means fewer side effects, more sustainable results, and outcomes that feel authentic rather than chemically induced.

THE EMOTIONAL AND PSYCHOLOGICAL DIMENSIONS

But perhaps the most important lesson I've learned is that true health optimization must address the emotional and psychological dimensions of wellness. I've seen too many patients whose physical symptoms improved with peptides and hormone optimization, only to plateau because we hadn't addressed the underlying emotional and mental factors that were contributing to their health issues.

Our bodies and minds are not separate entities—they're intimately connected through complex networks of hormones, neurotransmitters, and immune system signals. Chronic stress, unresolved trauma, negative thought patterns, and emotional imbalances can all manifest as physical symptoms and interfere with healing processes.

I remember one patient whose chronic pain and autoimmune symptoms didn't respond to any of our interventions until we discovered and addressed her history of childhood sexual abuse. The trauma had left her nervous system in a constant state of hypervigilance, triggering chronic inflammation and interfering with her body's natural healing mechanisms. It wasn't until we helped her process the trauma and teach her nervous system to feel safe again that her physical healing could begin.

This is why my approach now includes comprehensive assessment of emotional health, trauma history, stress patterns, and mental well-being. True healing requires us to address the whole person, not just their physical symptoms.

BUILDING A NEW MODEL OF MEDICINE

Today, at Viva La Skin in Myrtle Beach, we practice medicine differently. When patients come to see us, we don't just look at their chief complaint and current symptoms. We take time to understand their complete history—their genetics, their environment, their relationships, their stressors, their dreams and goals.

We use advanced testing to understand their unique biochemical needs, and we create personalized protocols that may include peptides, hormone optimization, nutritional support, stress management, and aesthetic treatments that help them look and feel their best.

But more than that, we see each patient as a unique individual worthy of comprehensive care. We take time to listen, to understand, and to create treatment plans that address their specific needs and goals. We're not just treating diseases—we're helping people optimize their lives.

This is the medicine of the future: personalized, preventative, regenerative, and focused on helping people thrive rather than just survive. It's medicine that respects the complexity of human beings and the sophisticated mechanisms by which our bodies heal and optimize themselves.

WHY THIS MATTERS NOW MORE THAN EVER

We're living in an unprecedented time in human history. Chronic diseases are epidemic. Mental health issues are skyrocketing. People are aging faster and dying younger than they should be. Traditional medicine, despite its many advances, is struggling to address these complex, multifaceted health challenges.

Meanwhile, the field of regenerative and integrative medicine is exploding with new discoveries and possibilities. We're learning more about the intricate connections between genetics, environment, lifestyle, and health. We're developing sophisticated tools like peptide therapy that can support the body's natural healing and optimization processes. We're beginning to understand how to address root causes rather than just managing symptoms.

But with this explosion of knowledge and possibilities comes confusion and misinformation. The internet is full of conflicting advice, unregulated products, and self-proclaimed experts who lack the training and experience to guide people safely through their health optimization journeys.

That's why qualified medical professionals need to step up and provide leadership in this field. That's why I wrote this book. People deserve accurate, science-based information from practitioners who understand the complexities of the human body and take responsibility for patient safety.

More than that, people deserve to know what's possible. They deserve to understand that feeling tired, gaining weight, losing mental clarity, and struggling with chronic health issues aren't just inevitable parts of aging. They're often signs that our bodies need support—support that modern integrative medicine, enhanced with cutting-edge tools like peptide therapy, can provide.

WHAT YOU'LL DISCOVER IN THIS BOOK

In the chapters that follow, I'll share everything I've learned about peptide therapy and integrative health optimization. You'll discover my comprehensive approach to assessing patients as whole human beings, not just collections of symptoms. You'll learn about the science behind peptides and how they can support everything from weight management and cognitive function to tissue repair and longevity.

You'll understand how peptides fit into a broader framework of health optimization that includes hormone balancing, nutritional support, stress management, and aesthetic treatments that help you look and feel your best. You'll see how this integrated approach is revolutionizing medicine and creating possibilities that were unimaginable just a few years ago.

But most importantly, you'll learn how to be an informed advocate for your own health. You'll understand what questions to ask potential providers, how to evaluate treatment options, and how to build a comprehensive approach to health optimization that addresses your unique needs and goals.

This isn't about quick fixes or miracle cures. It's about understanding your body, optimizing your health, and working with qualified practitioners who have the training, experience, and commitment to help you achieve your goals safely and effectively.

The transformation that's possible through integrative medicine and peptide therapy isn't just physical—it's emotional, mental, and spiritual. When you feel strong, energetic, and vital, every aspect of your life improves. Your relationships deepen, your work becomes more fulfilling, and you approach each day with confidence and enthusiasm.

You deserve to feel your best. You deserve to live your most optimal life. The tools and knowledge exist to make that possible. The question is: Are you ready to take the next step toward becoming the healthiest, most vibrant version of yourself?

The journey begins now.

CHAPTER 2
HOW I SEE THE WHOLE HUMAN

*"When someone walks into my clinic, I don't see
a diagnosis waiting to happen. I see a complete
human being with a unique story, complex
biology, and untapped potential for healing."*

TWENTY YEARS OF PRACTICING MEDICINE TAUGHT ME SOMETHING
that medical school never could: lab values and symptoms are just
the tip of the iceberg. Beneath the surface lies a complex web of factors
that determine whether someone thrives or merely survives. To truly
help people heal and optimize their health, we must see them as whole
human beings, not collections of symptoms or numbers on a test result.

This holistic perspective didn't develop overnight. It emerged
through years of watching patients whose "normal" lab values didn't
match their lived experiences, whose symptoms seemed to defy conventional explanations, and whose healing required us to address far
more than their physical complaints. Today, when I assess a patient

at Viva La Skin, I'm not just looking at their current symptoms—I'm exploring their complete human experience.

THE FIVE PILLARS OF HUMAN HEALTH

Through years of practice and thousands of patient interactions, I've identified five interconnected pillars that determine our overall health and vitality: physical, emotional, mental, spiritual, and genetic/environmental. True healing requires us to assess and address all five areas because they don't exist in isolation—they constantly influence and shape each other.

Think of these pillars like the foundation of a house. You might be able to shore up one or two weak areas temporarily, but if the foundation isn't solid across all pillars, the structure will eventually show signs of stress. This is why someone can eat perfectly, exercise regularly, and take all the right supplements, yet still feel exhausted and unwell if their emotional or spiritual health is compromised.

THE PHYSICAL PILLAR: BEYOND BASIC LAB WORK

When most people think about health assessment, they picture the physical pillar—blood tests, physical exams, diagnostic imaging. And yes, understanding someone's physical health is crucial. But the way I approach physical assessment goes far beyond checking boxes on a standard lab panel.

I'm looking at comprehensive hormone profiles, not just whether testosterone or estrogen fall within "normal" ranges, but whether they're optimized for that individual's age, lifestyle, and goals. I'm assessing inflammatory markers, nutrient status, metabolic function, sleep quality, and cellular energy production. I'm examining how their body processes and eliminates toxins, how efficiently they digest and absorb nutrients, and how well their various systems communicate with each other.

But even within the physical realm, I'm always asking deeper questions: Why is this person's inflammation elevated? What's causing their hormone imbalance? Why isn't their body producing energy efficiently? These "why" questions often lead me to the other pillars, because physical symptoms frequently have emotional, mental, or spiritual root causes.

THE EMOTIONAL PILLAR: WHERE FEELINGS BECOME PHYSICAL

Perhaps the most underestimated aspect of health assessment is the emotional pillar. In traditional medicine, we often dismiss emotional factors as secondary or separate from "real" medical issues. But the truth is that emotions create chemical reactions in our bodies. Chronic emotional stress, unresolved trauma, persistent anxiety, or deep-seated anger don't just affect our mood—they alter our physiology in profound ways.

When I assess emotional health, I'm exploring several key areas:

Past Trauma and Its Ongoing Impact: Traumatic experiences don't just live in our memories—they live in our bodies. I've seen patients whose chronic pain, autoimmune symptoms, or hormonal imbalances were directly linked to unprocessed trauma from years or even decades earlier.

I remember examining a patient, Lisa, a 34-year-old teacher who presented with severe chronic fatigue and mysterious pain throughout her body. Multiple specialists had run extensive tests, but everything came back normal. During my evaluation, she revealed that she had been sexually abused as a child. She had never connected her physical symptoms to her past trauma, but her body was essentially stuck in a state of hypervigilance, constantly preparing for danger that no longer existed.

Current Stress Patterns: How someone responds to daily stressors tells me a lot about their overall resilience and recovery capacity. Are they constantly overwhelmed by minor challenges? Do they have healthy coping mechanisms? Are they able to shift from stress to recovery mode?

Emotional Processing Abilities: Some people have learned healthy ways to process difficult emotions, while others tend to suppress, avoid, or become overwhelmed by their feelings. Those who struggle with emotional processing often develop physical symptoms as their bodies attempt to express what their minds cannot.

The key insight I've gained over the years is that emotions aren't just psychological experiences—they're biological events that trigger cascades of hormonal and immune system responses. Chronic negative emotions can suppress immune function, elevate inflammation, disrupt hormone production, and interfere with healing processes.

THE MENTAL PILLAR: HOW WE THINK AFFECTS HOW WE FEEL

Closely related to emotional health is mental health, but I consider them distinct pillars because they operate through different mechanisms. Mental health encompasses our thought patterns, belief systems, cognitive function, and psychological resilience.

When assessing mental health, I'm looking at several factors:

Cognitive Function: How clearly is this person thinking? Are they experiencing brain fog, memory issues, or difficulty concentrating? These symptoms can result from hormonal imbalances, nutrient deficiencies, sleep disorders, or chronic stress, but they significantly impact quality of life and need to be addressed.

Thought Patterns and Belief Systems: The stories we tell ourselves about our health, our capabilities, and our future have enormous power to influence our actual outcomes. Someone who believes they're destined to develop the same diseases as their parents may unconsciously make choices that fulfill that prophecy.

Sleep and Recovery: Mental health significantly impacts sleep quality, and poor sleep undermines both mental and physical health. I'm always exploring sleep patterns, dreams, and recovery quality as windows into someone's overall mental well-being.

THE SPIRITUAL PILLAR: PURPOSE, MEANING, AND CONNECTION

The spiritual pillar often surprises people because it's not something typically addressed in medical settings. But spiritual health—which I define as having a sense of purpose, meaning, and connection to something greater than oneself—is a crucial component of overall well-being.

Spiritual health doesn't necessarily mean religious belief, though it can include that. I'm talking about:

Sense of Purpose: People who feel their lives have meaning and direction tend to have better health outcomes, greater resilience, and longer lifespans. Conversely, those who feel disconnected from purpose often struggle with depression, anxiety, and physical symptoms that seem to have no clear cause.

Connection to Community: Humans are social beings, and our health suffers when we feel isolated or disconnected from others. Strong social connections support immune function, reduce inflammation, and provide crucial emotional support during challenging times.

I recall evaluating a patient, Michael, who had been struggling with depression and chronic fatigue for years. He had tried multiple medications and therapies with limited success. During my assessment, I discovered that he had been working in a corporate job that conflicted deeply with his values and sense of purpose. Once we addressed his spiritual health by helping him transition to work that felt meaningful, his depression lifted and his energy returned without any additional medical interventions.

THE GENETIC AND ENVIRONMENTAL PILLAR: UNDERSTANDING YOUR UNIQUE BLUEPRINT

The final pillar encompasses the genetic and environmental factors that influence health. This includes not just family history and inherited genetic variations, but also environmental exposures, lifestyle patterns, and epigenetic factors that determine how our genes are expressed.

Genetic Testing and Analysis: For patients who can afford it, I often recommend comprehensive genetic testing that looks at variations in genes related to hormone metabolism, detoxification, neurotransmitter function, and nutrient processing. For example, someone with MTHFR gene mutations may need specific forms of B vitamins and support for methylation processes.

Environmental Exposures: I explore both current and past environmental exposures that might be impacting health. This includes everything from mold exposure and chemical toxins to electromagnetic fields and chronic noise pollution.

HOW THE PILLARS INTERACT: THE CASE OF MARIA

To illustrate how these five pillars interact, let me share the story of a patient I evaluated—Maria, a forty-eight-year-old teacher who presented with a complex array of symptoms including chronic fatigue, weight gain, brain fog, and irregular menstrual cycles.

Physical Assessment: Maria's labs revealed low thyroid function, insulin resistance, elevated cortisol, and several nutrient deficiencies.

Traditional medicine would have likely prescribed thyroid medication and recommended diet and exercise.

Emotional Assessment: Maria revealed a history of childhood emotional abuse and a recent divorce that had left her feeling overwhelmed and anxious. She had been carrying enormous guilt about the impact of the divorce on her children.

Mental Assessment: Maria was experiencing significant brain fog and memory issues that were affecting her teaching performance. She had developed a pattern of negative self-talk and was convinced she was "falling apart" and would never feel normal again.

Spiritual Assessment: The divorce had left Maria feeling disconnected from her previous faith community, and she felt lost and without purpose beyond caring for her children.

Genetic/Environmental Assessment: Genetic testing revealed mutations affecting her ability to process certain B vitamins and detoxify estrogen metabolites. She had also been exposed to significant mold in her previous home.

THE INTEGRATED TREATMENT APPROACH

Rather than addressing each pillar separately, we created an integrated treatment plan that recognized how all five areas were interconnected:

Physical Interventions: We optimized her thyroid function, addressed her insulin resistance with specific peptides, and corrected her nutrient deficiencies with targeted supplementation based on her genetic variations.

Emotional Support: Maria began working with a trauma-informed therapist to process her childhood experiences and divorce. We also incorporated stress-reduction techniques and emotional regulation practices into her daily routine.

Mental Health: We used peptides that support cognitive function and neurotransmitter balance, while also helping Maria develop more positive thought patterns and realistic expectations for her healing journey.

Spiritual Reconnection: Maria began exploring new ways to connect with purpose and community, including volunteer work that felt meaningful and aligned with her values.

Environmental Optimization: We addressed the mold exposure through targeted detoxification protocols and helped Maria create a healthier living environment.

Within six months, Maria's transformation was remarkable. Her energy returned, her weight stabilized, her cognitive function improved dramatically, and her mood became more stable and positive. But more than any single symptom improvement, Maria felt like herself again—confident, capable, and excited about her future.

WHY THIS APPROACH MATTERS

This comprehensive, five-pillar approach to health assessment might seem complex or time-consuming, but it's actually the most efficient way to achieve lasting results. When we address only one or two pillars, people often experience temporary improvements that don't last. But when we support all five pillars simultaneously, the improvements tend to be more dramatic and sustainable.

This is particularly important when working with peptides and other advanced therapies. These powerful tools work best when the foundation of health is solid across all pillars. Someone who receives peptide therapy without addressing their emotional trauma, spiritual disconnection, or environmental toxins may see some improvements, but they won't achieve the full potential of what's possible.

Moreover, this approach empowers patients to become active participants in their own healing rather than passive recipients of treatments. When people understand how their thoughts, emotions, relationships, and environment influence their physical health, they can make informed choices that support their well-being in every area of life.

THE ART OF SEEING THE WHOLE PERSON

Learning to see people as whole human beings rather than collections of symptoms is both an art and a science. It requires medical knowledge, intuition, empathy, and the ability to hold space for complex, sometimes contradictory information. It means being willing to explore uncomfortable topics, to sit with uncertainty, and to acknowledge that healing often requires courage as much as chemistry.

But when we get it right—when we truly see and address the whole person—the results can be transformational. People don't just feel better physically; they often describe feeling more alive, more authentic, and more connected to themselves and others than they have in years.

This is the foundation upon which all effective treatments, including peptide therapy, must be built. Before we can optimize someone's biochemistry, we must understand their complete human experience. Only then can we create treatment plans that address not just their symptoms, but their deepest desire to feel fully alive and vital.

CHAPTER 3
WHAT ARE PEPTIDES AND WHY SHOULD YOU CARE?

"Peptides are like master keys that unlock your body's own healing and optimization potential."

I F YOU'VE MADE IT THIS FAR IN THE BOOK, YOU'VE HEARD ME mention peptides multiple times as powerful tools for health optimization. You might be wondering: what exactly are these compounds, how do they work, and why am I so excited about their potential? This chapter will give you everything you need to know about peptides—from the basic science to practical applications, safety considerations, and the regulatory landscape that makes them both promising and sometimes controversial.

Let me start with a simple truth: peptides aren't magic bullets or miracle cures. They're sophisticated biological tools that work by supporting and enhancing your body's natural processes. When used appropriately as part of a comprehensive health optimization strategy, they can help you achieve levels of vitality, performance, and well-being that might have seemed impossible with traditional medicine alone.

But here's what makes peptides truly revolutionary: they represent a fundamental shift in how we approach medicine. Instead of fighting against your body's natural processes with synthetic drugs that often come with significant side effects, peptides work with your body's existing systems to restore optimal function. They're like giving your cells a software update that helps them remember how to function at their peak.

WHAT ARE PEPTIDES, REALLY?

At their most basic level, peptides are short chains of amino acids—the same building blocks that make up proteins. Think of amino acids like letters in an alphabet. Proteins are like full sentences or paragraphs, while peptides are more like words or short phrases. These "molecular words" carry specific messages that tell your cells how to function.

Your body naturally produces thousands of different peptides, each with specific roles in regulating biological processes. They act as messengers, hormones, neurotransmitters, and growth factors. They control everything from how you build muscle and burn fat to how you sleep, think, heal from injuries, and age.

The peptides I use in my practice are either identical to ones your body already makes or synthetic versions designed to enhance specific biological functions. Unlike pharmaceutical drugs, which often work by blocking or artificially stimulating biological processes, peptides typically work by supporting and optimizing your body's existing systems.

Here's what makes peptides particularly fascinating: they're incredibly specific in their actions. While a pharmaceutical drug might affect multiple systems throughout your body (leading to side effects), a well-designed peptide can target very specific cellular processes with minimal impact on other systems. It's like having a precision tool rather than a sledgehammer.

THE EVOLUTION OF PEPTIDE SCIENCE

The history of peptide research is fascinating and relatively recent. The first peptide hormone, insulin, was discovered in 1922, but it wasn't until the 1950s and 1960s that scientists began to understand the broader role of peptides in biological processes. The real breakthrough came in the 1970s and 1980s when researchers discovered growth hormone-releasing hormone and other regulatory peptides.

What's exciting is that we're still in the early stages of understanding peptide potential. New peptides are being discovered regularly, and our understanding of how to use existing peptides is becoming more sophisticated. The field is advancing so rapidly that what seemed impossible just five years ago is now routine in practices like mine.

The development of synthetic peptides has been particularly revolutionary. Scientists can now create peptides that are more stable, more potent, or more specific than their natural counterparts. They can also create entirely new peptides designed to target specific biological processes that we want to optimize.

THE SCIENCE OF CELLULAR COMMUNICATION

To understand how peptides work, you need to understand cellular communication. Your body is essentially a vast communication network, with trillions of cells constantly sending and receiving messages. These messages coordinate everything from your heartbeat and breathing to your immune responses and tissue repair.

Peptides are part of this communication system. When a peptide reaches its target cell, it binds to specific receptors on the cell surface, like a key fitting into a lock. This binding triggers a cascade of events inside the cell that ultimately leads to the desired biological response.

For example, growth hormone-releasing peptides (GHRPs) bind to receptors in your pituitary gland and signal it to release more growth hormone naturally. This is fundamentally different from taking synthetic growth hormone, which bypasses your body's natural control mechanisms. The peptide works with your existing systems, while synthetic hormones often work against them.

This distinction is crucial for understanding why peptides often have fewer side effects than traditional medications. They're working with your body's natural processes rather than forcing artificial changes. Your body recognizes peptides as familiar molecules and responds accordingly, rather than treating them as foreign substances that need to be processed and eliminated.

THE REGULATORY LANDSCAPE: WHY PEPTIDES EXIST IN A GRAY AREA

Before we dive into specific peptides and their benefits, we need to address the elephant in the room: peptides exist in a complex regulatory environment that can be confusing for both patients and providers.

The FDA does not currently approve peptides for most of the uses I'll discuss in this chapter. This doesn't mean they're dangerous or ineffective—it means they haven't gone through the lengthy and expensive FDA approval process for these specific applications. Many peptides are available for "research purposes only," which allows qualified medical providers to use them with appropriate patients while staying within legal boundaries.

This regulatory situation creates both opportunities and challenges. On one hand, it allows innovative practitioners to offer cutting-edge treatments that might not otherwise be available for years. The FDA approval process can take 10-15 years and cost hundreds of millions of dollars, which means many promising compounds never make it to market because there's insufficient financial incentive for pharmaceutical companies to pursue approval.

On the other hand, this regulatory environment places the burden of due diligence on both providers and patients to ensure safety and efficacy. It requires us to be more vigilant about sourcing, dosing, monitoring, and patient selection than we might be with FDA-approved medications.

When I work with peptides in my practice, I follow several strict protocols:

- I only use peptides from reputable compounding pharmacies that provide certificates of analysis proving purity and potency
- I stay current with the latest research on safety and efficacy by reviewing scientific literature regularly
- I carefully screen patients to ensure they're appropriate candidates for specific peptides
- I monitor patients closely for both positive responses and potential side effects
- I maintain detailed records and communicate openly with patients about the regulatory status of these treatments
- I never make claims about peptides "treating" or "curing" specific diseases, as that would be inappropriate given their regulatory status

CATEGORIES OF PEPTIDES AND THEIR APPLICATIONS

There are hundreds of different peptides with various applications, but I'll focus on the categories I use most frequently in my practice and that have the strongest evidence base for safety and efficacy.

Growth Hormone-Releasing Peptides (GHRPs)

These peptides stimulate your pituitary gland to produce more growth hormone naturally. As we age, growth hormone production declines significantly, contributing to muscle loss, increased body fat, reduced energy, slower healing, and other signs of aging. By age 60, most people are producing only about 25% of the growth hormone they produced in their twenties.

Common GHRPs include:
- **Ipamorelin**: Known for being very clean with minimal side effects. It's selective for growth hormone release without significantly affecting cortisol or prolactin levels, making it one of the safest options for long-term use.
- **CJC-1295**: Often combined with other peptides for enhanced effects. It has a longer half-life than some other GHRPs, allowing for less frequent dosing.
- **Sermorelin**: One of the most studied and well-tolerated options. It's actually identical to the first 29 amino acids of naturally occurring growth hormone-releasing hormone.

Benefits may include:
- Improved muscle mass and strength
- Enhanced fat burning, especially around the midsection
- Better sleep quality and recovery
- Increased energy and vitality

- Improved skin quality and healing
- Enhanced cognitive function
- Better bone density
- Improved cardiovascular health markers

How I use them: I typically start patients on conservative doses and monitor their response carefully. These peptides work best when combined with proper nutrition, exercise, and sleep optimization. I often recommend taking them before bed, as this mimics the body's natural growth hormone release pattern.

The beauty of GHRPs is that they work with your body's natural feedback mechanisms. Unlike synthetic growth hormone, which can shut down your natural production, these peptides actually enhance your body's ability to produce growth hormone on its own.

Weight Management and Metabolic Peptides

These peptides target various aspects of metabolism, appetite regulation, and fat burning. They're particularly valuable for patients struggling with weight loss resistance or metabolic dysfunction.

GLP-1 Receptor Agonists: These peptides mimic hormones that regulate blood sugar and appetite. They've been game-changers for patients with insulin resistance, diabetes, and obesity. Originally developed for diabetes management, we've discovered they have profound effects on weight management and overall metabolic health.

Benefits include:

- Significant weight loss (I've seen patients lose 20-40 pounds sustainably)
- Improved insulin sensitivity and blood sugar control
- Reduced cravings and appetite regulation

- Better cardiovascular health markers
- Improved fatty liver disease
- Better sleep quality (often improved as weight normalizes)

The mechanism is fascinating: these peptides slow gastric emptying, increase satiety, and improve insulin sensitivity. But they also seem to affect the brain's reward pathways, reducing cravings for high-calorie, processed foods.

AOD-9604: A fragment of growth hormone that specifically targets fat metabolism without affecting growth hormone receptors. This means you get the fat-burning benefits without some of the other effects of growth hormone stimulation.

How I use them: Weight management peptides work best when combined with lifestyle modifications. I never use them as standalone treatments but rather as tools to help patients achieve and maintain healthy weight loss. The key is using them as part of a comprehensive program that includes nutrition education, exercise planning, and behavior modification.

Cognitive Enhancement Peptides

These peptides cross the blood-brain barrier and support various aspects of brain function. They're particularly valuable for patients dealing with brain fog, memory issues, or age-related cognitive decline.

The brain is one of the most peptide-rich organs in the body, with numerous peptide systems regulating everything from memory formation to mood stabilization. As we age, many of these systems become less efficient, leading to cognitive decline that many people accept as "normal aging" but which is actually preventable and often reversible.

Nootropic peptides include:

- **Noopept**: Supports memory, learning, and cognitive processing. It increases levels of brain-derived neurotrophic factor (BDNF), which is crucial for neuron health and the formation of new neural connections.
- **Dihexa**: Promotes the growth of new brain connections and has been shown to improve cognitive function in both healthy individuals and those with cognitive impairment.
- **Cerebrolysin**: A complex mixture of peptides that supports overall brain health and neuroplasticity. It's particularly valuable for people recovering from brain injuries or dealing with neuro-degenerative conditions.

Benefits may include:

- Improved memory and recall
- Enhanced focus and concentration
- Better mental clarity and processing speed
- Increased creativity and problem-solving abilities
- Protection against age-related cognitive decline
- Better mood stability
- Improved stress resilience

How I use them: Cognitive peptides work best when combined with other brain health strategies like optimized nutrition, regular exercise, stress management, and quality sleep. I often recommend them for professionals who need peak cognitive performance, students preparing for important exams, or anyone concerned about maintaining brain health as they age.

Tissue Repair and Healing Peptides

These peptides accelerate the body's natural healing processes and are particularly valuable for people with injuries, chronic pain, or slow healing.

BPC-157 (Body Protective Compound): Perhaps the most impressive healing peptide I've worked with. It accelerates healing of muscles, tendons, ligaments, bones, and even gastrointestinal tissue. The research on BPC-157 is remarkable—it seems to promote healing throughout the body by enhancing the formation of new blood vessels, protecting organs from damage, and accelerating tissue repair.

TB-500 (Thymosin Beta-4): Promotes tissue repair and reduces inflammation throughout the body. It's particularly effective for soft tissue injuries and has anti-inflammatory properties that can help with chronic pain conditions.

Benefits may include:
- Faster healing from injuries
- Reduced chronic pain and inflammation
- Improved gut health and digestive function
- Better recovery from workouts
- Enhanced overall tissue integrity
- Improved joint health
- Better wound healing

These peptides are particularly valuable for athletes, people with chronic pain conditions, or anyone dealing with slow healing from injuries or surgeries.

Anti-Aging and Longevity Peptides

These peptides target various aspects of the aging process, from cellular repair to immune function optimization.

Epitalon: Supports telomere length and cellular aging processes. Telomeres are the protective caps on chromosomes that shorten as we age. Epitalon may help maintain telomere length, potentially slowing cellular aging.

Thymalin: Supports immune system function by helping to regulate the thymus gland, which is crucial for immune health but shrinks as we age.

NAD+ precursors: Support cellular energy production and DNA repair. NAD+ levels decline significantly as we age, and restoring them may have profound anti-aging effects.

REAL-WORLD RESULTS: WHAT I'VE SEEN IN PRACTICE

Let me share some detailed examples of the transformations I've witnessed with peptide therapy:

James, 52, Executive: I evaluated a patient, James, a 52-year-old executive who presented with crushing fatigue, brain fog, and 30 pounds of stubborn belly fat. Despite eating well and exercising regularly, he felt like he was aging rapidly. His testosterone was on the lower end of normal, his growth hormone levels were nearly undetectable, and his inflammatory markers were elevated.

We started him on a protocol including growth hormone-releasing peptides (Ipamorelin and CJC-1295) and metabolic support peptides. We also optimized his sleep, addressed some nutrient deficiencies, and implemented stress management techniques.

Within four months, he had lost 25 pounds, his energy was back to levels he hadn't experienced in years, and his mental clarity was sharper than ever. His follow-up labs showed improved growth hormone levels, better inflammatory markers, and optimized hormone balance. But more importantly, he felt like himself again—confident, energetic, and ready to tackle new challenges.

Michelle, 45, Teacher: I worked with a patient, Michelle, a 45-year-old teacher who struggled with chronic pain from old injuries and digestive issues that had persisted for years. Traditional treatments had provided minimal relief. She had seen multiple specialists, tried various medications, and even had some surgical interventions, but nothing provided lasting improvement.

We used tissue repair peptides (BPC-157 and TB-500) along with gut-healing protocols and comprehensive nutritional support. Her pain levels dropped by 80% within three months, and her digestive symptoms completely resolved. She was able to return to activities she loved, including hiking and yoga, and her overall quality of life improved dramatically.

Robert, 60, Retiree: I evaluated a patient, Robert, a 60-year-old retiree who was concerned about cognitive decline and wanting to age as gracefully as possible. He had noticed increasing forgetfulness, difficulty with complex tasks, and general mental sluggishness. His father had developed Alzheimer's disease, and Robert was determined to do everything possible to maintain his cognitive health.

We implemented a comprehensive anti-aging protocol including cognitive enhancement peptides, growth hormone support, and longevity-focused compounds. We also optimized his nutrition, implemented a targeted exercise program, and addressed some sleep issues.

His memory and mental sharpness improved significantly, and he felt more energetic and vital than he had in decades. Follow-up cognitive testing showed improvements in multiple areas, and he reported feeling more confident about his mental abilities.

SAFETY CONSIDERATIONS AND POTENTIAL SIDE EFFECTS

While peptides generally have fewer side effects than traditional medications, they're not without risks. It's important to understand potential side effects and work with a qualified provider who can monitor your response carefully.

Potential side effects vary depending on the specific peptide but may include:

- **Injection site reactions**: Redness, swelling, itching, or bruising at injection sites. This is usually mild and temporary.
- **Temporary water retention**: Some peptides can cause mild fluid retention, especially when first starting.
- **Changes in appetite**: Weight management peptides obviously affect appetite, but other peptides may also influence hunger and satiety.
- **Sleep disturbances**: Some people experience changes in sleep patterns when starting peptides, though this usually resolves as the body adjusts.
- **Headaches or dizziness**: Particularly when starting or changing doses.
- **Hormonal fluctuations**: Since many peptides affect hormone production, some people may experience temporary hormonal adjustments.

More serious but rare side effects can include allergic reactions or interactions with other medications. This is why working with a qualified medical provider is essential. We carefully screen patients for contraindications, start with conservative doses, and monitor closely for any adverse reactions.

THE IMPORTANCE OF QUALITY AND SOURCING

One of the biggest challenges in peptide therapy is ensuring quality and purity. Because peptides aren't FDA-regulated for most applications, the market includes both high-quality, pharmaceutical-grade products and questionable compounds of unknown purity and potency.

I only work with reputable compounding pharmacies that:

- Provide certificates of analysis for every batch showing purity and potency
- Follow strict quality control procedures and Good Manufacturing Practices
- Use pharmaceutical-grade ingredients from reliable sources
- Maintain proper storage and handling protocols
- Have established track records and positive reputations in the medical community

The difference between high-quality and low-quality peptides can be dramatic, both in terms of effectiveness and safety. Poor-quality peptides may be contaminated, improperly stored, or significantly less potent than advertised. This is another reason why working with an experienced provider is crucial—we have established relationships with reliable suppliers and can ensure you're getting high-quality compounds.

HOW PEPTIDES FIT INTO A COMPREHENSIVE HEALTH STRATEGY

While I'm clearly enthusiastic about peptides, it's important to understand that they're not standalone solutions. They work best when integrated into a comprehensive health optimization strategy that includes:

Optimized Nutrition: Peptides can't overcome a poor diet. They work best when supported by high-quality nutrition that provides the building blocks for cellular repair and optimization. This means adequate protein intake, plenty of micronutrients, and avoiding foods that promote inflammation.

Regular Exercise: Many peptides enhance recovery and performance, but they're not substitutes for regular physical activity. Exercise and peptides work synergistically to promote health and vitality. The muscle-building and fat-burning effects of growth hormone-releasing peptides, for example, are much more pronounced when combined with appropriate exercise.

Quality Sleep: Sleep is when many of the body's repair and optimization processes occur. Peptides can support better sleep, but they work best when combined with good sleep hygiene. Growth hormone release, for instance, primarily occurs during deep sleep stages.

Stress Management: Chronic stress undermines the benefits of any health intervention. Peptides can help with stress resilience, but they're most effective when combined with stress management practices like meditation, yoga, or therapy.

Hormone Optimization: Many peptides work by influencing hormone production or sensitivity. They often work best when combined with comprehensive hormone optimization, including thyroid support, adrenal health, and sex hormone balance.

THE FUTURE OF PEPTIDE THERAPY

The field of peptide therapy is evolving rapidly, and I'm excited about what the future holds. New peptides are being discovered and studied constantly, and our understanding of how to use existing peptides is becoming more sophisticated.

I expect to see:

- **More targeted peptides for specific conditions**: Scientists are developing increasingly specific peptides that target particular biological pathways with even greater precision.
- **Better delivery methods**: While most peptides currently require injection, researchers are developing oral, nasal, and transdermal delivery methods that could make peptides more convenient to use.
- **Improved safety profiles**: As we gain more experience with peptides, we're learning how to optimize dosing and timing to maximize benefits while minimizing side effects.
- **Eventually, FDA approval for some peptides**: Some peptides will likely go through the formal FDA approval process for specific indications, which will increase mainstream acceptance and insurance coverage.
- **Integration into mainstream medicine**: As evidence continues to accumulate, I expect peptides to become more widely accepted and used in conventional medical practice.

MAKING AN INFORMED DECISION ABOUT PEPTIDES

If you're considering peptide therapy, here are the key questions you should ask any potential provider:

1. **What is your experience with peptides?** Look for providers who have been working with peptides for years and can provide specific examples of patient outcomes. Ask about their training and continuing education in this field.
2. **What is your source for peptides?** Ensure they work with reputable compounding pharmacies and can provide certificates of analysis. Be wary of providers who are vague about their sources or who use peptides from questionable suppliers.

3. **How do you determine dosing and protocols?** Avoid providers who use one-size-fits-all approaches or extremely aggressive dosing. Look for practitioners who individualize protocols based on your specific needs, goals, and response.

4. **What monitoring do you provide?** Ensure they plan to monitor your response through regular follow-ups, lab work when appropriate, and careful tracking of both benefits and side effects.

5. **How do peptides fit into your overall approach?** Look for providers who see peptides as part of a comprehensive health strategy, not as standalone treatments. They should also address nutrition, exercise, sleep, stress management, and other factors that influence health.

6. **What are the realistic expectations and timeline?** Be wary of providers who promise dramatic results quickly or who make unrealistic claims about what peptides can achieve.

THE BOTTOM LINE ON PEPTIDES

Peptides represent one of the most exciting frontiers in regenerative and anti-aging medicine. When used appropriately by qualified providers as part of a comprehensive health optimization strategy, they can help people achieve levels of vitality, performance, and well-being that might have seemed impossible just a few years ago.

However, they're not magic bullets, miracle cures, or substitutes for fundamental health practices. They're sophisticated tools that work best when integrated into a holistic approach to health that addresses all aspects of human well-being.

The key to success with peptides is finding a qualified provider who understands both the science and the art of peptide therapy, who prioritizes safety and quality, and who sees peptides as part of a larger strategy for helping you achieve your optimal health.

What excites me most about peptides is their potential to help people not just treat disease, but to truly optimize their health and achieve their full potential. As we continue to discover new peptides and refine our understanding of how to use them, I believe we're at the beginning of a revolution in how we approach human health and longevity.

In the next chapter, we'll explore how peptides fit into a comprehensive body optimization strategy that includes hormone balancing, nutrition, sleep optimization, and other tools for achieving peak human performance.

CHAPTER 4
YOUR BODY, OPTIMIZED

"True optimization isn't about taking the most advanced compound or following the latest biohacking trend. It's about creating synergy between all the systems that make you human."

Now that you understand what peptides are and how I approach patients as whole human beings, it's time to explore how these powerful compounds fit into a comprehensive body optimization strategy. This is where the art and science of regenerative medicine truly come together—creating personalized protocols that address not just your symptoms, but your deepest desire to feel fully alive and vital.

Over the years, I've learned that peptides work best when they're part of an integrated approach that includes hormone optimization, targeted nutrition, sleep enhancement, stress management, genetic insights, and even aesthetic treatments that help you look as good as you feel. It's not about adding more interventions—it's about creating intelligent synergies that amplify your results while minimizing complexity.

THE SYMPHONY OF OPTIMIZATION

Think of body optimization like conducting a symphony orchestra. Each system in your body is like a different section of musicians—the hormones are your string section, nutrition is your brass, sleep is your percussion, and peptides are like the conductor's baton, helping coordinate all the other sections to create beautiful music together.

When I work with patients on optimization protocols, I'm not just looking at individual lab values or isolated symptoms. I'm listening for the harmony between all these systems and identifying where we can create better coordination. Sometimes the issue isn't that any one system is "broken"—it's that they're not communicating effectively with each other.

I learned this lesson the hard way through my own personal health crisis. At 47, despite being a physician who understood the importance of health, I found myself in a terrible state. My BMI was in the obese category, I was prediabetic, slightly hypertensive, and had developed fatty liver disease. The fatigue, brain fog, and exhaustion were so severe that I could barely function. I remember going to CrossFit workouts and literally being unable to pick up weights that I should have been able to handle easily.

Here I was, a medical doctor, feeling absolutely terrible despite having "normal" lab values according to traditional standards. My labs read normal, but I felt completely abnormal. This disconnect between what the numbers said and how I actually felt was a wake-up call that changed my entire approach to medicine.

This integrated approach has evolved from years of seeing patients in hospital settings where complex medical conditions required me to understand how multiple systems interact, but more importantly, from my own personal transformation. A patient might present with heart failure, but their condition could be influenced by hormone imbalances, nutritional deficiencies, sleep disorders, and chronic stress. Treating just the heart without addressing these other factors would be like trying to fix a car by only looking at the engine while ignoring the transmission, fuel system, and electrical components.

My own health crisis forced me to look beyond traditional medicine's limitations and embrace the comprehensive approach I now use with my patients.

HORMONE OPTIMIZATION: THE FOUNDATION OF VITALITY

Before we can optimize anything else, we need to understand and balance your hormonal system. Hormones are chemical messengers that influence virtually every aspect of how you feel and function. When they're optimized, everything else becomes easier. When they're imbalanced, even the best nutrition and exercise programs will fall short of their potential.

The Major Players in Hormonal Health:

Thyroid Hormones: Often called the "master metabolic hormones," thyroid hormones control your energy production, body temperature, weight management, brain function, and mood. I frequently encounter patients whose thyroid function is "normal" according to standard lab ranges but suboptimal for their individual needs. Optimizing thyroid function often involves looking beyond just TSH and including Free T3, Free T4, Reverse T3, and thyroid antibodies.

Sex Hormones: Testosterone, estrogen, and progesterone don't just affect sexual function—they influence muscle mass, bone density, mood, cognitive function, cardiovascular health, and overall vitality. As we age, these hormones decline, but the rate and pattern of decline varies dramatically between individuals. Optimization often involves bioidentical hormone replacement, but the key is achieving physiologic levels that make you feel your best, not just bringing numbers into "normal" ranges.

Adrenal Hormones: Your adrenal glands produce cortisol, DHEA, and other hormones that help you manage stress and maintain energy throughout the day. Chronic stress, poor sleep, and inadequate nutrition can dysregulate these systems, leading to fatigue, anxiety, mood swings, and difficulty recovering from exercise or illness.

Growth Hormone and IGF-1: These hormones become increasingly important as we age, influencing muscle mass, fat distribution, bone density, skin quality, healing, and overall vitality. Rather than using synthetic growth hormone, which can shut down natural production, I prefer using growth hormone-releasing peptides that enhance your body's own production.

How Peptides Enhance Hormone Optimization

This is where peptides become particularly powerful. Instead of simply replacing hormones that have declined, peptides can help your body produce and utilize hormones more effectively. For example:

- Growth hormone-releasing peptides stimulate natural GH production
- Certain peptides can improve insulin sensitivity, helping your body use hormones more effectively
- Some peptides support adrenal function and stress resilience
- Others can enhance thyroid hormone conversion and utilization

I evaluated a patient, David, a 48-year-old engineer who presented with classic symptoms of hormonal decline—fatigue, brain fog, decreased libido, and difficulty maintaining muscle mass despite regular exercise. His hormone levels were technically "normal" but clearly suboptimal for his goals and expectations.

Rather than immediately starting hormone replacement, we began with a protocol that included growth hormone-releasing peptides, adrenal support compounds, and targeted nutrition. Within twelve weeks, his natural hormone production had improved significantly, his energy was restored, and his body composition had changed dramatically. We achieved optimization by enhancing his body's own hormone production rather than replacing it entirely.

David's case reminded me of my own experience when I finally sought help at Unity Health for comprehensive testing. Despite feeling terrible, my testosterone levels were "low normal"—technically within range but clearly not optimal for how I wanted to feel and function. When we addressed this with a low dose of testosterone replacement as part of a comprehensive protocol, it was one of the key pieces that helped restore my vitality.

TARGETED NUTRITION: FUELING YOUR OPTIMIZATION

Nutrition is the foundation upon which all other optimization strategies are built. You can have the most advanced peptide protocols and perfectly balanced hormones, but if your nutrition isn't supporting your goals, you'll never achieve your full potential.

However, when I talk about nutrition for optimization, I'm not referring to generic dietary advice or the latest trending diet. I'm talking about precision nutrition based on your individual biochemistry, genetic variations, health goals, and lifestyle demands.

The Optimization Nutrition Framework

Protein Optimization: Adequate protein intake becomes even more critical when using peptides, especially growth hormone-releasing compounds and tissue repair peptides. Your body needs amino acid building blocks to synthesize new proteins, build muscle, and repair tissues. I typically recommend 0.8-1.2 grams of high-quality protein per pound of body weight for people on optimization protocols.

Micronutrient Density: Many people are unknowingly deficient in key vitamins and minerals that support hormone production, cellular energy, and peptide effectiveness. Common deficiencies I see include vitamin D, B vitamins, magnesium, zinc, and omega-3 fatty acids. These aren't just "nice to have"—they're essential cofactors for the biological processes we're trying to optimize.

Meal Timing and Frequency: When you eat can be as important as what you eat, especially when using certain peptides. Growth hormone-releasing peptides, for example, work best when taken on an empty stomach, typically before bed. Some weight management peptides are most effective when timed around meals to optimize their appetite and metabolic effects.

Anti-Inflammatory Foods: Chronic inflammation undermines every aspect of optimization. I emphasize foods that naturally reduce inflammation—fatty fish, leafy greens, berries, nuts, seeds, and high-quality olive oil—while minimizing inflammatory foods like processed sugars, refined grains, and industrial seed oils.

Genetic-Based Nutrition: For patients who can afford comprehensive genetic testing, we can identify specific nutritional needs based on genetic variations. Someone with MTHFR mutations might need methylated B vitamins, while someone with APOE4 variants might benefit from specific dietary modifications to support brain health.

I worked with a patient, Sandra, a 52-year-old attorney who had been struggling with energy crashes, sugar cravings, and weight gain around her midsection. Her diet was technically "healthy"—she ate organic foods, avoided processed junk, and followed general dietary guidelines—but she wasn't seeing results.

Genetic testing revealed several variations affecting her ability to process carbohydrates and metabolize certain fats. We modified her nutrition plan based on these insights and combined it with targeted peptides for metabolic support. Within eight weeks, her energy was stable throughout the day, her cravings had disappeared, and she had lost fifteen pounds while gaining muscle mass.

SLEEP OPTIMIZATION: THE ULTIMATE RECOVERY TOOL

Sleep is when most of your body's repair, recovery, and optimization processes occur. Growth hormone is primarily released during deep sleep. Memory consolidation happens during REM sleep. Cellular cleanup and toxin elimination accelerate during sleep. If your sleep isn't optimized, no amount of peptides, hormones, or perfect nutrition will deliver their full potential.

Yet sleep optimization goes far beyond just getting eight hours per night. Quality matters more than quantity, and there are specific strategies that can dramatically enhance sleep's restorative power.

The Architecture of Optimal Sleep:

Sleep Timing: Your circadian rhythm is controlled by light exposure, meal timing, and temperature fluctuations. Going to bed and waking up at consistent times helps synchronize these rhythms. I often recommend using blue light blocking glasses in the evening and getting bright light exposure early in the morning.

Sleep Environment: Your bedroom should be cool (65-68°F), completely dark, and quiet. Many people underestimate how much ambient light and noise affect sleep quality. Room-darkening shades, white noise machines, or earplugs can make a significant difference.

Pre-Sleep Routine: What you do in the hour before bed dramatically affects sleep quality. This includes when you take certain peptides, what you eat, how you manage stress, and how you prepare your mind and body for rest.

Sleep Stages: Optimal sleep includes adequate time in both deep sleep (for physical recovery) and REM sleep (for mental recovery). Some peptides can actually enhance sleep quality by promoting deeper, more restorative sleep stages.

How Peptides Can Enhance Sleep:

Certain peptides have remarkable effects on sleep quality:

- Growth hormone-releasing peptides often improve deep sleep stages
- Some cognitive enhancement peptides can improve REM sleep and dream quality
- Specific peptides designed for stress management can help calm an overactive nervous system
- Tissue repair peptides often enhance the restorative aspects of sleep

I evaluated a patient, Marcus, a 45-year-old executive who complained of waking up tired despite getting seven to eight hours of sleep nightly. Sleep tracking revealed that he was spending very little time in deep sleep stages, likely due to chronic stress and elevated cortisol levels.

We implemented a protocol that included stress-management peptides, evening cortisol-lowering supplements, and growth hormone-releasing peptides timed to enhance natural sleep architecture. Within a month, his deep sleep had nearly doubled, he was waking up refreshed, and his daytime energy and cognitive performance had improved dramatically.

STRESS MANAGEMENT: THE HIDDEN OPTIMIZATION FACTOR

Chronic stress is the enemy of optimization. It elevates cortisol, which interferes with hormone production, disrupts sleep, promotes inflammation, and undermines the effectiveness of every other intervention. Yet most people dramatically underestimate how much stress affects their physiology.

The Physiology of Stress and Optimization:

When you're chronically stressed, your body prioritizes survival over optimization. Resources get diverted from muscle building, tissue repair, immune function, and hormone production toward immediate stress response. This is why someone can do everything "right" with their diet, exercise, and supplements but still feel terrible if they're not managing stress effectively.

Stress Management Strategies That Work:

Mindfulness and Meditation: Regular meditation practice has been shown to lower cortisol, improve heart rate variability, enhance immune function, and even support healthy gene expression. Even ten to fifteen minutes daily can make a significant difference.

Breathwork: Specific breathing techniques can rapidly shift your nervous system from a fight-or-flight state to a rest-and-digest mode. Box breathing, also known as coherent breathing, and other techniques can be powerful tools for immediate stress relief.

Movement and Exercise: Regular physical activity is one of the most effective stress management tools, but the type and intensity matter. Moderate exercise reduces stress, while excessive high-intensity exercise can increase cortisol levels.

Social Connection: Strong relationships and social support are among the most powerful predictors of health and longevity. Loneliness and social isolation create chronic stress that undermines optimization efforts.

How Peptides Support Stress Resilience:

Certain peptides can enhance your ability to handle stress:

- Some peptides support healthy cortisol patterns and adrenal function
- Others can improve heart rate variability and nervous system balance
- Cognitive enhancement peptides often improve stress resilience and mental clarity under pressure
- Sleep-supporting peptides help ensure you're getting the recovery you need to handle daily stressors

GENETIC INSIGHTS: YOUR PERSONAL OPTIMIZATION BLUEPRINT

One of the most exciting developments in optimization medicine is our ability to understand individual genetic variations that affect how you respond to different interventions. Your genes influence everything from how you metabolize medications and supplements to how you respond to exercise and nutrition.

Key Genetic Variations for Optimization:

MTHFR Mutations: Affect your ability to process folate and B vitamins, which are crucial for hormone production, neurotransmitter synthesis, and cellular energy production.

APOE Variants: Influence brain health, cardiovascular risk, and how you respond to different types of fats in your diet.

COMT Variations: Affect how you break down dopamine and norepinephrine, influencing stress resilience, cognitive function, and response to certain supplements.

CYP450 Variations: Determine how quickly you metabolize various medications and compounds, affecting dosing and timing recommendations.

I worked with a patient, Jennifer, a 41-year-old marketing director who had tried multiple optimization protocols with limited success. She exercised regularly, ate well, and had tried various supplements, but nothing seemed to move the needle on her energy or body composition.

Genetic testing revealed that she had variations affecting her ability to methylate B vitamins and process certain compounds. We modified her supplement protocol to include methylated vitamins and adjusted her peptide timing based on her genetic variations. Within six weeks, she experienced the energy and results she had been seeking for years.

Jennifer's case was particularly meaningful to me because it mirrored my genetic discoveries. When I finally had comprehensive testing done, I discovered I had MTHFR and COMT gene mutations that were significantly affecting my ability to process B vitamins and handle stress. I also found I was severely vitamin D deficient—despite living in sunny South Carolina and thinking I got adequate sun exposure.

These genetic insights completely changed my supplementation approach. Instead of generic vitamins, I started taking 5-methyltetrafolate (the active form of folate that people with MTHFR mutations can use) and high-dose vitamin D. The difference was remarkable and helped me understand why standard approaches hadn't been working for me.

EXERCISE AND RECOVERY: MAXIMIZING YOUR INVESTMENT

Exercise is crucial for optimization, but more isn't always better. The key is finding the right type, intensity, and frequency of exercise for your individual goals, recovery capacity, and lifestyle demands. Peptides can significantly enhance both exercise performance and recovery, but they work best when integrated into a thoughtful exercise program.

Optimization-Focused Exercise Principles:

Progressive Overload: Your body adapts to demands placed on it, so gradually increasing challenge is essential for continued improvement. This applies whether your goal is strength, endurance, mobility, or body composition.

Recovery Priority: Growth and adaptation happen during recovery, not during exercise itself. This means managing exercise volume and intensity to match your recovery capacity.

Movement Quality: Perfect form and movement patterns are more important than heavy weights or intense cardio. Poor movement patterns can lead to injuries that derail optimization efforts.

Variety and Periodization: Your body adapts to repetitive stress, so varying exercises, intensities, and training focuses helps prevent plateaus and overuse injuries.

How Peptides Enhance Exercise and Recovery:

Different peptides can support various aspects of exercise and recovery:

- Growth hormone-releasing peptides enhance muscle growth and fat loss from exercise
- Tissue repair peptides accelerate recovery from workouts and reduce injury risk
- Cognitive enhancement peptides can improve focus and mind-muscle connection during training
- Anti-inflammatory peptides help manage exercise-induced inflammation

AESTHETIC INTEGRATION: LOOKING AS GOOD AS YOU FEEL

This might surprise you, but aesthetic treatments can be an important part of comprehensive optimization. When you look better, you feel more confident, which affects your stress levels, motivation, and overall quality of life. Moreover, many aesthetic treatments work synergistically with optimization protocols to enhance results.

Aesthetic Treatments That Support Optimization:

Skin Health: Healthy, vibrant skin often reflects internal health. Treatments that support collagen production, cellular turnover, and skin hydration can enhance the effects of internal optimization protocols.

Body Contouring: Sometimes despite optimal nutrition and exercise, stubborn fat deposits or loose skin can affect how you feel about your body. Strategic aesthetic treatments can help you achieve the physical appearance that matches your internal improvements.

Hair Health: Hair loss can significantly affect confidence and quality of life. Certain peptides and treatments can support hair growth and thickness.

Facial Optimization: As we age, facial volume loss and skin changes can make us look tired or older than we feel. Strategic treatments can help ensure your appearance matches your vitality.

At Viva La Skin, we integrate aesthetic treatments with optimization protocols because we understand that how you look affects how you feel, and how you feel affects how you look. It's not vanity—it's comprehensive wellness.

CREATING YOUR PERSONAL OPTIMIZATION PROTOCOL

The key to successful optimization is creating a personalized protocol that addresses your individual needs, goals, lifestyle, and preferences. This isn't about following someone else's program—it's about creating a sustainable approach that works for your unique situation.

My transformation is the perfect example of how this integrated approach works in practice. Once I identified my hormone imbalances, genetic mutations, and nutritional deficiencies, I didn't just address each issue in isolation. I created a comprehensive protocol that included:

- **Hormone optimization** with low-dose testosterone replacement that brought my levels to optimal rather than just "normal"
- **Genetic-based supplementation** with 5-methyltetrafolate and high-dose vitamin D to address my specific mutations and deficiencies
- **Peptide therapy** including BPC-157 for gut healing and to address chronic calf injuries that had been limiting my exercise performance

- **Targeted nutrition** with an elimination diet followed by the systematic introduction of anti-inflammatory foods
- **Structured exercise** with a regimented workout routine designed to complement my other interventions

The results were nothing short of transformational. I went from having a "dad bod" with obesity, prediabetes, and fatty liver to what I can only describe as "Greek statue status." But more importantly than the physical transformation, I felt like myself again—energetic, mentally sharp, and physically capable.

This experience completely changed my perspective on medicine and ignited my passion for helping others achieve similar transformations. If I could go from feeling terrible despite being a physician who "should have known better" to achieving optimal health and vitality, then anyone can do it with the right approach and guidance.

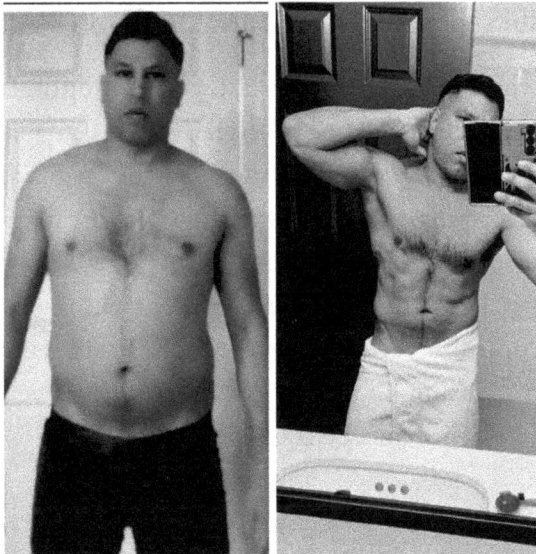

The Optimization Assessment Process:

Comprehensive Lab Work: Beyond basic blood chemistry, this includes comprehensive hormone panels, inflammatory markers, nutrient levels, and metabolic markers.

Lifestyle Assessment: Understanding your sleep patterns, stress levels, exercise habits, nutrition patterns, and life demands.

Goal Clarification: What does optimization mean to you? More energy? Better body composition? Enhanced cognitive performance? Improved sexual health? Slower aging?

Genetic Testing: When appropriate and affordable, genetic insights can guide more precise interventions.

Monitoring and Adjustment: Optimization is an ongoing process that requires regular monitoring and protocol adjustments based on your response and changing goals.

THE SYNERGISTIC EFFECT: WHY INTEGRATION MATTERS

When all these elements work together—optimized hormones, targeted nutrition, quality sleep, effective stress management, appropriate exercise, and strategic peptide use—the results are often greater than the sum of the parts. This is the synergistic effect that makes comprehensive optimization so powerful.

I evaluated a patient, Thomas, a 55-year-old business owner who wanted to optimize every aspect of his health and performance. Rather than focusing on any single intervention, we created an integrated protocol that addressed all the factors I've discussed in this chapter.

His hormone levels were optimized through a combination of bioidentical hormone replacement and growth hormone-releasing peptides. His nutrition was personalized based on genetic testing and metabolic analysis. We optimized his sleep environment and timing. He implemented stress management practices that fit his lifestyle. His exercise program was designed to complement his peptide protocols and recovery capacity.

The transformation was remarkable. Within six months, Thomas had the energy and vitality of someone twenty years younger, his body composition had improved dramatically, his cognitive performance was sharper than ever, and he felt more confident and capable than he had in decades. But more importantly, he felt like the best version of himself—physically, mentally, and emotionally.

THE FUTURE OF PERSONALIZED OPTIMIZATION

As our understanding of human biology continues to advance, optimization protocols will become increasingly personalized and precise. We're moving toward a future where we can predict how someone will respond to specific interventions based on their genetics, microbiome, metabolic profile, and other individual factors.

Artificial intelligence will help us identify patterns and optimize protocols in ways that would be impossible for any individual practitioner to achieve. Wearable technology will provide real-time feedback on how interventions are affecting sleep, stress, recovery, and performance.

But despite all these technological advances, the fundamental principles will remain the same: optimization requires a comprehensive approach that addresses the whole person, not just isolated symptoms or systems.

YOUR NEXT STEPS TOWARD OPTIMIZATION

If you're ready to begin your own optimization journey, the most important step is finding a qualified practitioner who understands how all these elements work together. Look for someone who:

- Takes a comprehensive approach to assessment and treatment
- Has experience with peptide therapy and hormone optimization
- Understands the importance of nutrition, sleep, stress management, and exercise
- Can provide ongoing monitoring and protocol adjustments
- Sees optimization as a process, not a destination

Remember, optimization isn't about perfection—it's about progress. It's about feeling better today than you did yesterday and better next month than you do today. It's about aging gracefully while maintaining vitality, performance, and quality of life.

The tools and knowledge exist to help you achieve levels of health and vitality that previous generations could only dream of. The question isn't whether optimization is possible—it's whether you're ready to commit to the process of becoming the best version of yourself.

CHAPTER 5
THE REGENERATIVE REVOLUTION

*"We're not just treating disease anymore—
we're rewriting the rules of what it means to
age, to heal, and to thrive as human beings."*

SOMETHING EXTRAORDINARY IS HAPPENING IN MEDICINE right now. We're witnessing the emergence of a completely new paradigm that's challenging everything we thought we knew about health, aging, and human potential. This isn't just another medical trend or fad—it's a fundamental shift toward regenerative, personalized, and optimization-focused healthcare that puts patients in control of their own biology.

I call it the Regenerative Revolution, and peptides are at the forefront of this transformation. But to understand why peptides are so significant, you need to understand the broader context of how medicine is evolving and why traditional approaches are no longer adequate for the health challenges we face today.

THE OLD PARADIGM: DISEASE-FOCUSED MEDICINE

For the past century, medicine has been primarily focused on diagnosing and treating disease. This approach has been remarkably successful for acute conditions—infections, injuries, surgical emergencies, and other immediate threats to health. If you have a heart attack, need emergency surgery, or develop pneumonia, modern medical technology can literally save your life.

But this disease-focused model has significant limitations when it comes to the chronic health challenges that most people face today. It's reactive rather than proactive, waiting for problems to develop rather than preventing them. It treats symptoms rather than addressing root causes. It sees the body as a collection of separate systems rather than an integrated whole.

Most importantly, it doesn't help people optimize their health and vitality—it just helps them manage illness and dysfunction.

During my years practicing in hospital settings, I saw the limitations of this model every day. I treated patients with diabetes who were managing their blood sugar but weren't truly healthy. I worked with people suffering from chronic fatigue who had "normal" lab values but felt terrible. I encountered countless individuals who were technically disease-free but far from optimal.

But it wasn't until I became one of those patients myself that I truly understood the profound limitations of traditional medicine. At 47, despite being a physician, I found myself obese, prediabetic, hypertensive, with fatty liver disease, crushing fatigue, and brain fog so severe I could barely function. I was working out at CrossFit but couldn't even pick up the weights I should have been able to handle.

The most frustrating part? According to traditional medicine, I was "fine." My labs were "normal." Every specialist I saw told me my numbers looked good. But I felt absolutely terrible, and no one in the traditional medical system seemed to understand the disconnect between what the lab values said and how I actually felt.

This personal health crisis forced me to look beyond conventional medicine and discover the regenerative approaches that ultimately saved my health and my life. When I finally found providers who understood optimization rather than just disease management, everything changed.

The traditional model asks: "What's wrong with you, and how do we fix it?"

The regenerative model asks: "How can we help you achieve your optimal health and vitality?"

THE NEW PARADIGM: REGENERATIVE AND OPTIMIZATION MEDICINE

The Regenerative Revolution represents a fundamental shift toward a new model of healthcare that's:

- **Proactive Rather Than Reactive**: Instead of waiting for disease to develop, we focus on optimizing health and preventing problems before they occur.
- **Root Cause Focused**: Rather than just managing symptoms, we identify and address the underlying factors that contribute to health issues.
- **Personalized and Precision-Based**: We recognize that every individual is unique and requires customized approaches based on their genetics, biochemistry, lifestyle, and goals.
- **Integration and Systems-Thinking**: We understand that the body is an interconnected system where everything affects everything else.
- **Patient-Empowered**: We see patients as active participants in their own health optimization rather than passive recipients of treatments.

- **Technology-Enhanced**: We leverage cutting-edge tools like genetic testing, advanced diagnostics, wearable technology, and innovative therapies like peptides to achieve better outcomes.

THE BIOHACKING MOVEMENT: CITIZENS TAKING CONTROL

One of the driving forces behind the Regenerative Revolution is the biohacking movement—a growing community of individuals who are taking active control of their own biology and health optimization. Biohackers use data, technology, and experimental approaches to enhance their physical and cognitive performance.

This movement includes everyone from Silicon Valley executives using continuous glucose monitors to optimize their diet, to athletes experimenting with recovery technologies, to everyday people tracking their sleep and stress levels to improve their quality of life.

What's remarkable about the biohacking community is their willingness to experiment, measure, and iterate. They're not content to accept "normal" as optimal. They're constantly asking: "How can I feel better, perform better, and age more gracefully?"

This mindset has accelerated the adoption of innovative therapies like peptides, advanced hormone optimization, targeted nutrition, and other regenerative approaches. Biohackers are often the early adopters who prove that these interventions work, paving the way for broader acceptance in mainstream medicine.

The Democratization of Health Optimization

What used to be available only to elite athletes or wealthy individuals is becoming accessible to anyone who's committed to optimizing their health. Advanced lab testing, genetic analysis, peptide therapy, and other optimization tools are more available and affordable than ever before.

This democratization is empowering people to take control of their health rather than relying solely on traditional healthcare systems. They're becoming informed consumers who understand their biology and make proactive choices about their health.

LONGEVITY SCIENCE: REDEFINING WHAT'S POSSIBLE

Another major driver of the Regenerative Revolution is the explosion of longevity science, research focused on understanding and slowing the aging process itself. Scientists are discovering that aging isn't just an inevitable decline but a complex biological process that can be influenced and potentially slowed.

Key Discoveries in Longevity Science:

Cellular Senescence: We now understand that aging is partly caused by the accumulation of senescent cells—cells that have stopped dividing but haven't died. These "zombie cells" secrete inflammatory compounds that accelerate aging. Researchers are developing interventions to clear these cells and restore tissue function.

Telomere Biology: Telomeres are protective caps on chromosomes that shorten as we age. Maintaining telomere length may slow cellular aging and extend healthy lifespan.

NAD+ Metabolism: NAD+ is a crucial molecule for cellular energy production and DNA repair. NAD+ levels decline significantly with age, but restoring them may have profound anti-aging effects.

Protein Quality Control: Our cells have sophisticated systems for maintaining protein quality, but these systems become less efficient with age. Supporting these mechanisms may slow aging and prevent age-related diseases.

Hormetic Stress: Controlled stresses like exercise, fasting, and heat

PEPTIDE PRESCRIPTION

exposure can strengthen our cellular repair mechanisms and extend lifespan.

Peptides play important roles in many of these longevity pathways. Some peptides support telomere maintenance, others enhance cellular repair mechanisms, and still others optimize hormone production that declines with age.

THE TECHNOLOGY REVOLUTION: TOOLS FOR OPTIMIZATION

The Regenerative Revolution is being accelerated by technological advances that give us unprecedented insight into our biology and the ability to make precise interventions.

Advanced Diagnostics: We can now measure biomarkers that weren't even known to exist a few decades ago. Comprehensive hormone panels, inflammatory markers, nutritional status, genetic variations, and metabolic function can all be assessed with remarkable precision.

Genetic Testing: For less than the cost of a weekend getaway, you can now understand your genetic predispositions, medication sensitivities, nutritional needs, and optimization opportunities.

Wearable Technology: Devices that track sleep, heart rate variability, stress levels, activity, and even blood sugar are providing real-time feedback on how lifestyle choices affect health and performance.

Artificial Intelligence: AI is helping identify patterns in health data that would be impossible for humans to detect, leading to more personalized and effective interventions.

Precision Manufacturing: Compounding pharmacies can now create customized medications, including peptides, tailored to individual needs and specifications.

I worked with a patient, Karen, a 49-year-old engineer who exemplified this technology-enabled approach to optimization. She used

70

continuous glucose monitoring to optimize her diet, tracked her sleep and recovery with wearable devices, and used genetic testing to guide her supplement choices.

When we added peptide therapy to her optimization protocol, she was able to track in real-time how the peptides affected her sleep quality, recovery metrics, and metabolic markers. This data-driven approach allowed us to fine-tune her protocol for maximum effectiveness.

PEPTIDES: THE PERFECT TOOL FOR THE NEW PARADIGM

Peptides represent the perfect intersection of cutting-edge science and personalized medicine. They embody everything that the Regenerative Revolution stands for:

Precision Medicine: Peptides can target very specific biological pathways and processes, allowing for precise interventions tailored to individual needs.

Working With Biology: Unlike pharmaceutical drugs that often work against the body's natural processes, peptides support and enhance existing biological systems.

Customizable: Peptide protocols can be highly customized based on individual goals, genetics, lifestyle, and response patterns.

Minimal Side Effects: Because peptides work with natural processes, they typically have fewer side effects than traditional medications.

Measurable Results: The effects of peptides can often be tracked through objective measures like lab work, body composition, sleep quality, and performance metrics.

Proactive Rather Than Reactive: Peptides can be used for optimization and prevention, not just treating existing problems.

THE INTEGRATION OF TRADITIONAL AND ALTERNATIVE APPROACHES

One of the most exciting aspects of the Regenerative Revolution is how it's bringing together the best of traditional medicine with innovative approaches that were previously considered "alternative."

Evidence-Based Alternative Medicine: Practices like acupuncture, meditation, herbal medicine, and nutritional therapy are being studied with rigorous scientific methods, validating their effectiveness and helping us understand how they work.

Functional Medicine: This approach focuses on identifying and addressing root causes of health issues rather than just treating symptoms. It considers factors like nutrition, stress, sleep, environmental exposures, and genetics in understanding health and disease.

Integrative Medicine: This combines conventional medical treatments with evidence-based complementary approaches, providing patients with the full spectrum of healing options.

Lifestyle Medicine: Recognition that lifestyle factors—nutrition, exercise, sleep, stress management, and social connections—are often more powerful than medications for preventing and treating chronic diseases.

As a physician who has worked in both traditional hospital settings and integrative practice, I see tremendous value in combining the best of all approaches. Emergency medicine and acute care remain crucial, but for optimization and chronic disease prevention, we need the broader toolkit that regenerative medicine provides.

THE BUSINESS OF HEALTH OPTIMIZATION

The Regenerative Revolution isn't just changing how we practice medicine—it's creating entirely new business models and economic opportunities around health optimization.

Direct-Pay Medicine: Many optimization-focused practitioners are moving away from insurance-based models toward direct-pay relationships with patients. This allows for longer appointment times, more comprehensive assessments, and innovative treatments that may not be covered by insurance.

Concierge Medicine: High-end medical practices that provide comprehensive, personalized care with unlimited access to physicians and cutting-edge treatments.

Wellness Centers and Med Spas: Facilities that combine medical expertise with spa-like environments, offering everything from IV therapy and peptide treatments to aesthetic procedures and wellness coaching.

Online Health Platforms: Telemedicine and digital health platforms are making optimization services accessible to people who don't have local providers offering these approaches.

Health Coaching: Professional coaches who help people implement lifestyle changes and optimization strategies, bridging the gap between medical care and daily life.

This shift toward market-based healthcare is empowering both providers and patients. Providers can focus on delivering value and results rather than navigating insurance bureaucracies. Patients can invest in their health proactively rather than just paying for disease treatment.

GLOBAL TRENDS DRIVING THE REVOLUTION

The Regenerative Revolution is being driven by several global trends that are converging to create unprecedented opportunities for health optimization:

Aging Population: As life expectancy increases, people want to maintain vitality and quality of life throughout their extended lifespans. Simply living longer isn't enough—people want to live better.

Rising Healthcare Costs: Traditional healthcare is becoming increasingly expensive and often ineffective for chronic conditions. People are looking for alternatives that provide better value and outcomes.

Information Access: The internet has democratized access to health information, empowering people to become educated consumers who demand better options.

Technology Adoption: Younger generations are comfortable using technology to track and optimize their health, driving demand for data-driven approaches.

Lifestyle-Related Disease: The epidemic of diabetes, obesity, heart disease, and other lifestyle-related conditions is creating demand for prevention-focused approaches.

Performance Culture: In our competitive society, people are constantly looking for ways to enhance their performance, productivity, and capabilities.

CHALLENGES AND CONTROVERSIES

The Regenerative Revolution isn't without its challenges and controversies. As with any paradigm shift, there are legitimate concerns that need to be addressed:

Regulatory Issues: Many innovative treatments, including peptides, exist in regulatory gray areas. This creates both opportunities and risks for patients and providers.

Quality Control: The rapid growth of the optimization industry has attracted some providers who may lack adequate training or use questionable practices.

Cost and Access: Many optimization approaches are expensive and not covered by insurance, potentially creating disparities in access to these advances.

Overpromising: Some practitioners make exaggerated claims about what optimization can achieve, leading to unrealistic expectations.

Safety Concerns: Any powerful intervention carries risks, and the long-term effects of some optimization approaches aren't fully understood.

Scientific Rigor: Not all optimization practices are backed by robust scientific evidence, and there's a need for more research in many areas.

As a medical professional, I believe these challenges are best addressed through education, ethical practice, continued research, and appropriate regulation that protects patients while allowing innovation to flourish.

THE ROLE OF MEDICAL PROFESSIONALS

The Regenerative Revolution is creating new roles and responsibilities for medical professionals. We're no longer just diagnosticians and treatment providers—we're becoming health coaches, optimization consultants, and partners in our patients' wellness journeys.

My transformation from a sick, tired physician to someone who achieved optimal health has completely changed how I practice medicine. When I tell patients about the possibilities of optimization, I'm not just sharing theoretical knowledge—I'm sharing what I've personally experienced and achieved.

When I went from obese and prediabetic to having the body composition and energy levels of someone half my age, I realized that if a 47-year-old physician who had let his health deteriorate so dramatically could achieve such a transformation, then anyone can do it with the right approach and guidance. This personal experience gives me credibility and passion that I could never have gained from textbooks or medical training alone.

The Evolution of Medical Practice:

From Treatment to Optimization: Moving beyond fixing problems to helping people achieve their full potential.

From Protocol-Driven to Personalized: Customizing approaches based on individual needs rather than following standardized protocols.

From Episodic to Continuous: Developing ongoing relationships focused on long-term optimization rather than just addressing immediate problems.

From Isolated to Integrative: Working with other professionals—nutritionists, fitness experts, health coaches, mental health providers—to address all aspects of health.

From Reactive to Proactive: Focusing on prevention and optimization rather than waiting for problems to develop.

This evolution requires medical professionals to continuously update their knowledge, develop new skills, and embrace approaches that may not have been part of their traditional training.

THE PATIENT OF THE FUTURE

The Regenerative Revolution is also changing what it means to be a patient. People are becoming active participants in their health optimization rather than passive recipients of medical care.

Characteristics of the Optimized Patient:

Educated and Informed: They understand their biology and make informed decisions about their health.

Data-Driven: They track biomarkers, symptoms, and outcomes to optimize their approaches.

Proactive: They invest in prevention and optimization rather than waiting for problems to develop.

Collaborative: They work in partnership with healthcare providers rather than simply following orders.

Experimental: They're willing to try new approaches and adjust based on results.

Long-Term Focused: They think about health as a lifelong investment rather than just addressing immediate concerns.

This shift requires patients to take more responsibility for their own health, but it also empowers them to achieve results that weren't possible under the traditional model.

LOOKING FORWARD: THE FUTURE OF MEDICINE

As I look toward the future, I see the Regenerative Revolution continuing to accelerate and transform how we approach human health and potential. Several trends are likely to shape this evolution:

Personalized Medicine: Treatments will become increasingly customized based on individual genetics, microbiome, metabolic profiles, and other personal factors.

Preventive Focus: Healthcare systems will gradually shift toward prevention and optimization rather than just disease treatment.

Technology Integration: AI, wearable devices, and other technologies will provide real-time health monitoring and personalized recommendations.

Longevity Medicine: Treating aging itself will become a medical specialty, with interventions designed to extend both lifespan and healthspan.

Global Access: Technology will help democratize access to optimization approaches, making them available to people regardless of geographic location.

Evidence Base: More research will validate optimization approaches and help us understand how to use them most effectively.

YOUR ROLE IN THE REVOLUTION

The Regenerative Revolution isn't something that's happening to you—it's something you can actively participate in and benefit from. Whether you're dealing with specific health challenges or simply want to optimize your vitality and performance, you have unprecedented opportunities to take control of your biology.

How to Become Part of the Revolution:

Educate Yourself: Learn about your biology, health optimization principles, and available interventions.

Track Your Data: Use wearable devices, lab testing, and other tools to understand your current health status and track improvements.

Find Qualified Providers: Work with medical professionals who understand optimization approaches and can guide you safely through the process.

Experiment and Iterate: Be willing to try new approaches, measure results, and adjust based on what works for your unique situation.

Think Long-Term: Invest in your health proactively rather than waiting for problems to develop.

Stay Current: The field is evolving rapidly, so stay informed about new developments and opportunities.

The tools, knowledge, and opportunities exist today to help you achieve levels of health, vitality, and performance that previous generations could only dream of. The question isn't whether the Regenerative Revolution will continue—it's whether you're ready to be part of it.

I know this is possible because I've lived it myself. When I started my optimization journey at 47, feeling terrible despite being a physician, I could never have imagined the transformation that was possible. Going from obese and prediabetic to optimal health wasn't just about changing my body—it changed my entire life and career trajectory.

That transformation taught me that if I can do it, so can you. Every patient I work with now benefits not just from my medical training and expertise, but from my personal experience of what's truly possible when we embrace this new paradigm of medicine.

Peptides represent just one tool in this revolutionary approach to health and human optimization. But when used as part of a comprehensive, personalized strategy, they can help you unlock your body's full potential and live the vibrant, optimized life you deserve.

The revolution is here. The question is: Are you ready to join it?

CHAPTER 6
AESTHETICS MEETS LONGEVITY

"True beauty isn't about looking younger—
it's about looking like the healthiest, most
vibrant version of yourself at any age."

THERE'S A PROFOUND CONNECTION BETWEEN HOW WE LOOK and how we feel that goes far deeper than vanity or superficial concerns. When you look in the mirror and see someone who appears vital, healthy, and confident, it affects your mood, your energy, your relationships, and your entire approach to life. Conversely, when you see someone who looks tired, aged, or unhealthy, it can create a downward spiral that affects every aspect of your well-being.

This is why I've come to believe that aesthetic medicine and longevity medicine aren't separate fields—they're two sides of the same coin. True aesthetics isn't about chasing youth or conforming to artificial beauty standards. It's about optimizing your appearance to reflect your internal vitality and helping you feel confident in your own skin at every stage of life.

At Viva La Skin, we've created what I believe is the future of aesthetic medicine—an integrated approach that combines advanced cosmetic treatments with comprehensive health optimization. We don't just help people look better; we help them feel better, function better, and live better. And we do it by addressing the root causes of aging rather than just treating the symptoms.

THE PSYCHOLOGY OF APPEARANCE AND SELF-PERCEPTION

The relationship between appearance and self-perception is complex and deeply ingrained in human psychology. Multiple studies have shown that when people feel good about how they look, they have higher self-esteem, greater confidence, improved mood, and better social interactions. This isn't vanity—it's basic human psychology.

But here's what's interesting: the improvements in confidence and mood that come from looking better often translate into better health behaviors. When people feel good about themselves, they're more likely to exercise regularly, eat well, manage stress effectively, and take care of their overall health. This creates a positive feedback loop where looking better leads to feeling better, which leads to behaving better, which leads to being healthier.

My own transformation illustrated this perfectly. As I went from having what I can only describe as a "dad bod" to achieving what people now call "Greek statue status," the changes weren't just physical. My confidence soared, my energy increased, my relationships improved, and my entire approach to life became more positive and optimistic. Looking like the healthy, vital person I had become on the inside completely transformed how I moved through the world.

This experience taught me that aesthetic improvements aren't separate from health optimization—they're an integral part of it. When we help someone look their best, we're also helping them become their best.

THE BIOLOGICAL BASIS OF AGING AND APPEARANCE

To understand how aesthetics and longevity intersect, we need to understand what actually causes the visible signs of aging. It's not just the passage of time—it's a complex interplay of biological processes that affect both how we look and how we function.

The Major Factors in Aesthetic Aging:

Collagen Degradation: Collagen is the protein that gives skin its structure, firmness, and elasticity. Starting in our twenties, we lose about 1% of our collagen each year. This loss accelerates with sun exposure, stress, poor nutrition, and hormonal changes.

Cellular Senescence: As cells age, they become senescent—essentially "zombie cells" that stop functioning properly but don't die. These cells secrete inflammatory compounds that accelerate aging throughout the body, including the skin.

Hormonal Decline: The decrease in growth hormone, sex hormones, and thyroid hormones that occurs with age directly affects skin quality, muscle mass, fat distribution, and overall vitality.

Glycation: When excess sugar in the bloodstream binds to proteins like collagen, it creates advanced glycation end products (AGEs) that make tissues stiff and dysfunctional.

Oxidative Stress: Free radicals damage cells throughout the body, including skin cells, leading to premature aging and decreased function.

Volume Loss: As we age, we lose fat and bone volume in specific

PEPTIDE PRESCRIPTION

areas, particularly the face, which creates the hollow, aged appearance that many people associate with getting older.

The remarkable thing about these aging processes is that they can all be influenced through the same interventions we use for health optimization. Peptides, hormone optimization, targeted nutrition, stress management, and other longevity strategies don't just help you feel better—they help you look better too.

THE INSIDE-OUT APPROACH TO AESTHETICS

Traditional aesthetic medicine often focuses on surface-level treatments—injecting fillers to restore volume, using lasers to resurface skin, or performing surgical procedures to lift and tighten tissues. While these approaches can certainly be effective, they're addressing symptoms rather than causes.

The inside-out approach we use at Viva La Skin starts with optimizing the biological processes that determine how you age. When you support your body's natural collagen production, optimize your hormones, reduce inflammation, and enhance cellular repair processes, you don't just slow aging—you can actually reverse many signs of aging while preventing future damage.

How Internal Optimization Enhances Appearance:

Peptide Therapy for Aesthetic Enhancement: Many of the peptides we use for health optimization also have remarkable aesthetic benefits:

- Collagen-stimulating peptides can improve skin texture, firmness, and elasticity

- Growth hormone-releasing peptides enhance muscle tone and reduce fat in stubborn areas
- Hair growth peptides can restore thickness and coverage
- Wound healing peptides can improve skin repair and reduce scarring

Hormone Optimization for Aesthetic Benefits: Balanced hormones don't just improve how you feel—they dramatically affect how you look:

- Optimal testosterone levels enhance muscle mass and reduce abdominal fat
- Balanced estrogen supports skin hydration and collagen production
- Thyroid optimization improves skin texture and hair quality
- Growth hormone support enhances overall body composition

Nutrition for Beauty: The foods you eat become the building blocks for your skin, hair, and overall appearance:

- Adequate protein provides amino acids for collagen synthesis
- Antioxidants protect against oxidative damage
- Healthy fats support hormone production and skin health
- Proper hydration maintains skin plumpness and elasticity

Sleep and Stress Management for Aesthetics: Poor sleep and chronic stress accelerate aging through multiple mechanisms:

- Cortisol elevation breaks down collagen and impairs skin repair
- Poor sleep disrupts growth hormone release, which is crucial for tissue repair
- Stress creates inflammation that accelerates all aging processes

I worked with a patient, Rebecca, a 52-year-old real estate agent who was considering extensive cosmetic surgery to address what she felt was rapid aging. Instead of immediately pursuing surgical options, we implemented a comprehensive optimization protocol that included peptide therapy, hormone balancing, targeted nutrition, and stress management.

Within six months, her skin quality had improved dramatically, she had lost 20 pounds of stubborn fat, her energy was restored, and her overall appearance was so transformed that people regularly commented that she looked ten years younger. She achieved results that were superior to what surgery could have provided, but through optimizing her biology rather than fighting against it.

THE SYNERGY OF INTERNAL AND EXTERNAL TREATMENTS

While I'm a strong advocate for the inside-out approach, I also recognize that combining internal optimization with targeted external treatments can achieve results that neither approach could accomplish alone. This is the synergistic model we use at Viva La Skin.

Advanced Aesthetic Treatments That Complement Optimization:

Regenerative Skin Treatments: Procedures like microneedling, radiofrequency, and laser treatments can stimulate collagen production and improve skin texture. When combined with peptides and proper nutrition that support collagen synthesis, the results are enhanced and longer-lasting.

Strategic Volume Restoration: Carefully placed dermal fillers can restore facial volume and create more youthful contours. When combined with optimization protocols that improve skin quality and body composition, the results look more natural and integrated.

Body Contouring: Sometimes despite optimal nutrition and exercise, genetic factors or previous weight fluctuations can leave stubborn fat deposits or loose skin. Advanced body contouring treatments can address these issues while optimization protocols ensure the best possible healing and results.

Hair Restoration: Hair loss can significantly affect confidence and self-perception. Combining advanced hair restoration techniques with peptides and hormone optimization often produces superior results compared to either approach alone.

The key is using external treatments strategically to enhance and complement the improvements achieved through internal optimization, rather than using them to fight against ongoing aging processes.

THE ROLE OF CONFIDENCE IN HEALTH AND LONGEVITY

There's growing scientific evidence that confidence and positive self-perception actually contribute to better health outcomes and increased longevity. People who feel good about themselves tend to:

- Take better care of their health
- Have stronger immune function
- Experience less stress-related illness
- Maintain more active social lives
- Pursue challenging goals and experiences

This creates a powerful argument for aesthetic treatments as legitimate health interventions. When we help someone feel more confident and positive about their appearance, we're not just improving their quality of life—we may actually be extending their lifespan.

My own experience bears this out. As my physical transformation progressed and I began to look like the healthy, vital person I was becoming internally, my confidence and outlook on life improved dramatically. I found myself taking on new challenges, pursuing opportunities I might have avoided, and generally approaching life with more energy and optimism.

This psychological transformation was just as important as the physical changes, and it contributed to my overall health and well-being in ways that went far beyond appearance.

THE FUTURE OF INTEGRATED AESTHETIC MEDICINE

I believe we're moving toward a future where the distinction between aesthetic medicine and health optimization will largely disappear. Instead of separate specialties focused on either health or appearance, we'll have integrated practices that recognize the fundamental connection between how we look and how we feel.

Emerging Trends in Aesthetic Medicine:

Precision Aesthetics: Using genetic testing, advanced imaging, and biomarker analysis to create highly personalized aesthetic treatment plans.

Regenerative Treatments: Therapies that harness the body's own healing and repair mechanisms to restore youthful function and appearance.

Preventive Aesthetics: Starting aesthetic interventions earlier to prevent aging rather than just treating existing signs of aging.

Holistic Integration: Combining aesthetic treatments with nutrition, exercise, stress management, and other lifestyle factors for comprehensive results.

Technology Enhancement: Using artificial intelligence, advanced imaging, and other technologies to optimize treatment planning and outcomes.

CREATING YOUR INTEGRATED AESTHETIC STRATEGY

If you're interested in an integrated approach to aesthetics and longevity, here are the key principles to consider:

Start with Optimization: Before pursuing any external treatments, optimize your internal biology through proper nutrition, exercise, sleep, stress management, and appropriate supplementation or peptide therapy.

Address Root Causes: Rather than just treating symptoms of aging, identify and address the underlying factors that are accelerating the aging process.

Think Long-Term: Focus on interventions that will continue to provide benefits over time rather than quick fixes that require constant maintenance.

Work with Qualified Providers: Find practitioners who understand both aesthetic medicine and health optimization, and who can create integrated treatment plans.

Monitor and Adjust: Use objective measures to track your progress and adjust your approach based on results.

Maintain Realistic Expectations: Remember that the goal is to look like the healthiest, most vibrant version of yourself, not to look like someone else or to stop aging entirely.

THE VIVA LA SKIN MODEL

At Viva La Skin, we've created what I believe is the ideal model for integrated aesthetic and longevity medicine. Our approach includes:

Comprehensive Assessment: We evaluate not just your aesthetic concerns, but your overall health, hormone levels, nutritional status, and lifestyle factors.

Personalized Protocols: Based on your assessment, we create customized treatment plans that address both internal optimization and external enhancement.

Advanced Treatments: We offer the latest in both aesthetic procedures and optimization therapies, including peptide treatments, hormone optimization, and regenerative procedures.

Ongoing Support: We provide continuous monitoring, adjustment, and support to ensure you achieve and maintain your goals.

Education and Empowerment: We help you understand the science behind our approaches so you can make informed decisions about your care.

The results we achieve with this integrated approach consistently exceed what either aesthetic treatments or health optimization could accomplish alone. Our patients don't just look better—they feel better, function better, and approach life with renewed confidence and vitality.

THE PSYCHOLOGY OF AGING GRACEFULLY

One of the most important aspects of integrated aesthetic medicine is helping people develop a healthy relationship with aging. The goal isn't to stop aging or to look decades younger than your chronological age. The goal is to age gracefully while maintaining your vitality, confidence, and quality of life.

This means accepting the natural changes that come with age while taking proactive steps to optimize how you age. It means enhancing your natural features rather than trying to look like someone else. It means focusing on health and vitality rather than just appearance.

When people embrace this approach, they often find that they not only look better, but they feel more authentic and confident in their own skin. They're not fighting against aging—they're optimizing the aging process to ensure they look and feel their best at every stage of life.

YOUR AESTHETIC AND LONGEVITY JOURNEY

Whether you're dealing with specific aesthetic concerns or simply want to optimize how you age, the integrated approach offers the best path forward. By addressing both internal optimization and external enhancement, you can achieve results that are natural, long-lasting, and deeply satisfying.

The key is finding providers who understand this integrated approach and who can help you create a personalized strategy based on your unique needs, goals, and circumstances. This isn't about following someone else's program—it's about creating an approach that helps you become the best version of yourself.

Remember, true beauty and vitality come from the inside out. When you optimize your health, manage stress effectively, nourish your body properly, and address any underlying imbalances, your external appearance will naturally reflect your internal vitality.

But don't underestimate the power of looking your best to help you feel your best. When you're confident in your appearance, you approach life differently. You take better care of yourself, pursue opportunities more aggressively, and generally live with more energy and optimism.

This is the future of aesthetic medicine—an integrated approach that recognizes the profound connection between how we look and how we feel, and that uses cutting-edge science to help people achieve both aesthetic and health goals simultaneously.

Your journey toward optimal health and appearance starts with a single decision—the decision to stop accepting "normal" as optimal and to start pursuing the vitality and confidence you deserve. The tools, knowledge, and treatments exist to help you achieve remarkable results. The question is: are you ready to begin?

CHAPTER 7
BECOMING THE CEO OF YOUR HEALTH

"Your health is your most valuable asset, and no one should care about it more than you. It's time to stop being a passive patient and start being the CEO of your own well-being."

THROUGHOUT THIS BOOK, I'VE SHARED THE SCIENCE BEHIND peptides, the power of integrated health optimization, and the transformative potential of regenerative medicine. Now it's time to talk about the most important aspect of this entire journey: your role as the leader of your own health.

The traditional medical model has conditioned us to be passive patients who wait for problems to develop, then hand over responsibility to doctors who tell us what's wrong and prescribe solutions. But the optimization approach requires a completely different mindset—one where you take active ownership of your health, make informed decisions about your care, and work in partnership with qualified providers to achieve your goals.

This shift from patient to CEO of your health is perhaps the most crucial element in achieving the kind of transformation I've experienced personally and witnessed in hundreds of patients. When you take ownership of your health and commit to optimization rather than just disease management, everything changes.

The Mindset Shift: From Sick Care to Self Care

The first step in becoming the CEO of your health is understanding the fundamental difference between sick care and self care. The traditional medical system is actually a sick care system—it's designed to diagnose and treat illness, not to help healthy people become optimally healthy.

This isn't a criticism of traditional medicine. Emergency departments, surgical interventions, and acute care are absolutely crucial when you're dealing with serious illness or injury. But if your goal is to feel your best, perform at your peak, and age gracefully, you need to think beyond the sick care model.

Sick Care Mindset vs. CEO Mindset

Sick Care: "I'll deal with health issues if and when they arise"
CEO Mindset: "I invest in my health proactively to prevent problems and optimize performance"

Sick Care: "My doctor is responsible for my health"
CEO Mindset: "I'm responsible for my health, and I work with qualified advisors to achieve my goals"

Sick Care: "Normal lab values mean I'm healthy"
CEO Mindset: "I want to feel optimal, not just normal"

Sick Care: "I'll take whatever medication my doctor prescribes"
CEO Mindset: "I want to understand my options and make informed decisions about my care"

Sick Care: "Aging and declining health are inevitable"
CEO Mindset: "I can influence how I age and maintain vitality throughout my life"

My own transformation from a sick, tired physician to someone with optimal health perfectly illustrates this mindset shift. When I was operating from a sick care mindset, I accepted that feeling terrible was just part of being in my forties and having a demanding career. I thought my "normal" lab values meant I was fine, despite feeling anything but fine.

It wasn't until I shifted to a CEO mindset—taking ownership of my health, seeking out qualified advisors who understood optimization, and committing to the process of becoming my best self—that everything changed.

TAKING INVENTORY: WHERE ARE YOU NOW?

Just like any CEO needs to understand their company's current situation before making strategic decisions, you need to take honest inventory of your current health status. This goes beyond just getting an annual physical or basic lab work—it means comprehensive assessment of all the factors that influence your health and vitality.

Physical Assessment:

- Comprehensive lab work including hormones, inflammatory markers, nutrient levels, and metabolic markers

- Body composition analysis (not just weight, but muscle mass, fat percentage, and distribution)
- Cardiovascular fitness and strength assessment
- Sleep quality and patterns
- Energy levels throughout the day

Mental and Emotional Assessment:

- Stress levels and coping mechanisms
- Cognitive function (memory, focus, mental clarity)
- Mood stability and emotional resilience
- Sense of purpose and life satisfaction
- Relationship quality and social support

Lifestyle Assessment:

- Nutrition quality and patterns
- Exercise habits and physical activity
- Sleep hygiene and recovery practices
- Stress management techniques
- Environmental factors (living conditions, work environment, toxin exposure)

Goals and Vision Assessment:

- What does optimal health mean to you?
- What specific outcomes are you seeking?
- What timeline is realistic for your goals?
- What are you willing to invest (time, energy, resources) in your health?

This comprehensive assessment gives you the baseline data you need to make informed decisions about your health optimization journey.

FINDING YOUR HEALTH OPTIMIZATION TEAM

One of the biggest mistakes people make when pursuing health optimization is trying to do it alone or working with providers who don't understand the comprehensive approach required for true optimization. Just as successful CEOs surround themselves with knowledgeable advisors and specialists, you need to build a team of qualified professionals who can guide you through this process.

Essential Team Members for Health Optimization:

Primary Optimization Provider: This should be a physician or qualified practitioner who understands integrative medicine, peptide therapy, hormone optimization, and comprehensive health assessment. This person serves as your "quarterback," coordinating your overall strategy and monitoring your progress.

Specialized Practitioners: Depending on your needs, this might include endocrinologists, functional medicine doctors, nutritionists, fitness experts, mental health professionals, or aesthetic providers.

Testing and Monitoring Resources: Access to comprehensive lab testing, genetic analysis, body composition assessment, and other monitoring tools.

Support Network: Family, friends, health coaches, or support groups that understand and encourage your optimization journey.

QUESTIONS TO ASK POTENTIAL PROVIDERS

Finding qualified providers for health optimization can be challenging because this field is relatively new and not all practitioners have the necessary knowledge and experience. Here are the essential questions you should ask any potential provider:

Experience and Training Questions:

- How long have you been working with peptides and optimization protocols?
- What specific training do you have in peptide therapy, hormone optimization, and integrative medicine?
- Can you provide examples of patient transformations you've facilitated?
- How do you stay current with developments in this rapidly evolving field?

Approach and Philosophy Questions:

- How do you assess patients for optimization protocols?
- Do you take a comprehensive approach that includes lifestyle factors, not just supplements or medications?
- How do you personalize treatments based on individual needs and goals?
- What role do you expect me to play in my own health optimization?

Safety and Quality Questions:

- Where do you source your peptides and how do you ensure quality?
- Can you provide certificates of analysis for the compounds you use?
- How do you monitor patients for both benefits and potential side effects?
- What safety protocols do you follow?

Practical Questions:

- What does your assessment process involve?
- How often will you monitor my progress?
- What are realistic expectations for results and timeline?
- What are the costs involved and what payment options do you offer?

Red Flags to Avoid:

- Providers who make unrealistic promises or guarantee specific results
- Those who use one-size-fits-all approaches without comprehensive assessment
- Anyone who can't clearly explain their sourcing and quality control procedures
- Providers who dismiss the importance of lifestyle factors
- Those who seem more focused on selling products than optimizing your health

UNDERSTANDING YOUR OPTIONS

As the CEO of your health, you need to understand the full spectrum of options available for optimization. This knowledge empowers you to make informed decisions and avoid being limited by any single provider's preferred approaches.

Peptide Therapy Options:

- Growth hormone-releasing peptides for anti-aging and body composition
- Weight management peptides for metabolic optimization
- Cognitive enhancement peptides for mental performance
- Tissue repair peptides for healing and recovery
- Longevity peptides for cellular health

Hormone Optimization Approaches:

- Bioidentical hormone replacement therapy
- Natural hormone support through nutrition and lifestyle
- Targeted supplementation for hormone precursors
- Peptides that enhance natural hormone production

Advanced Testing and Monitoring:

- Comprehensive hormone panels
- Genetic testing for personalized insights
- Advanced imaging for body composition
- Continuous glucose monitoring for metabolic optimization
- Heart rate variability monitoring for stress assessment

Lifestyle Optimization Strategies:

- Personalized nutrition based on genetic and metabolic factors
- Targeted exercise programs for your specific goals
- Sleep optimization techniques and technologies
- Stress management and resilience training
- Environmental optimization (air, water, light, EMF)

CREATING YOUR PERSONAL OPTIMIZATION PLAN

With comprehensive assessment data and a qualified team in place, you can create a personalized optimization plan that addresses your unique needs and goals. This plan should be dynamic and evolve based on your progress and changing circumstances.

Key Elements of an Effective Optimization Plan:

Clear Goals and Metrics: Define specific, measurable outcomes you want to achieve. Instead of "feeling better," specify goals like "increase energy levels so I can work out intensely 5 days per week" or "improve cognitive function so I can focus for 3+ hours without fatigue."

Prioritized Interventions: Start with the most impactful interventions first. Usually this means addressing fundamental lifestyle factors (sleep, nutrition, exercise) before adding advanced therapies like peptides.

Implementation Timeline: Create a realistic timeline for implementing different aspects of your plan. Trying to change everything at once often leads to overwhelm and failure.

Monitoring Schedule: Establish regular check-ins and testing to track progress and make adjustments as needed.

Budget Considerations: Understand the costs involved and prioritize interventions based on both impact and affordability.

Lifestyle Integration: Ensure your plan fits realistically into your life and responsibilities. The best plan is useless if you can't actually follow it.

Let me share how this worked in my own transformation. After my comprehensive assessment revealed hormone imbalances, genetic mutations, and nutritional deficiencies, I created a prioritized plan:

Phase 1 (Months 1-2): Address basic deficiencies with vitamin D and methylated B vitamins, begin low-dose testosterone replacement, implement elimination diet

Phase 2 (Months 3-4): Add BPC-157 for gut healing and injury repair, establish consistent workout routine, optimize sleep environment

Phase 3 (Months 5-6): Fine-tune nutrition based on elimination diet results, add targeted supplements based on genetic testing, increase exercise intensity

This phased approach allowed me to implement changes gradually while monitoring what was working and what needed adjustment.

MONITORING PROGRESS AND MAKING ADJUSTMENTS

As the CEO of your health, you need robust systems for tracking progress and making data-driven decisions about your optimization strategy. This goes beyond just "feeling better"—you need objective measures that can guide your decisions.

Key Metrics to Track:

Objective Health Markers:

- Laboratory values (hormones, inflammatory markers, metabolic markers)
- Body composition changes (muscle mass, fat percentage, visceral fat)
- Physical performance measures (strength, endurance, flexibility)
- Sleep quality metrics (duration, efficiency, deep sleep percentage)
- Heart rate variability and stress indicators

Subjective Well-being Measures:

- Energy levels throughout the day
- Cognitive performance (focus, memory, mental clarity)
- Mood stability and emotional resilience
- Libido and sexual function
- Overall life satisfaction and quality of life

Functional Assessments:

- Work performance and productivity
- Exercise capacity and recovery
- Stress tolerance and resilience
- Social relationships and interactions

Regular monitoring allows you to identify what's working, what isn't, and what needs to be adjusted. This is crucial because optimization is not a one-time intervention—it's an ongoing process that requires continuous refinement.

INVESTMENT THINKING: UNDERSTANDING THE TRUE COST OF HEALTH

As the CEO of your health, you need to think about health expenses as investments rather than costs. This perspective shift is crucial for making decisions that serve your long-term interests rather than just minimizing short-term expenses.

Traditional Healthcare Costs vs. Optimization Investment:

Most people spend thousands of dollars per year on health insurance premiums, copays, medications, and treatments for chronic conditions. Yet they hesitate to invest in optimization approaches that could prevent many of these problems.

Consider the real costs of poor health:

- Lost productivity and earning potential due to fatigue and brain fog
- Increased medical expenses for chronic conditions
- Reduced quality of life and missed experiences
- Potential long-term care costs due to accelerated aging
- The psychological and emotional costs of feeling suboptimal

When you calculate these true costs, investment in optimization often provides exceptional return on investment, both financially and in terms of quality of life.

Making Smart Investment Decisions:

Start with High-Impact, Low-Cost Interventions: Basic lab testing, genetic analysis, and lifestyle optimization often provide the biggest return on investment.

Prioritize Based on Your Specific Needs: If you have severe hormone imbalances, hormone optimization might be your highest priority. If you have gut issues, peptides for digestive health might provide the most benefit.

Consider Long-Term Value: Interventions that provide ongoing benefits (like learning stress management techniques) often have better long-term value than those requiring continuous expense.

Invest in Knowledge and Skills: Learning about nutrition, exercise, and health optimization provides lifelong value that compounds over time.

NAVIGATING THE REGULATORY LANDSCAPE

As the CEO of your health, you need to understand the regulatory environment surrounding optimization treatments, particularly peptides. This knowledge helps you make informed decisions and work safely with qualified providers.

Key Regulatory Considerations:

FDA Status: Most peptides used for optimization are not FDA-approved for these specific applications. This doesn't mean they're dangerous, but it does mean you need to work with knowledgeable providers who understand how to use them safely.

Compounding Pharmacy Requirements: Ensure any peptides you use come from reputable compounding pharmacies that follow proper quality control procedures and can provide certificates of analysis.

Medical Supervision: Peptide therapy should always be conducted under qualified medical supervision, with appropriate monitoring and safety protocols.

Legal Compliance: Make sure your provider is operating within appropriate legal boundaries and following professional standards.

Understanding these factors helps you avoid questionable providers and ensure you're receiving safe, high-quality care.

BUILDING LONG-TERM SUCCESS HABITS

Sustainable health optimization isn't about short-term interventions—it's about building habits and systems that support long-term vitality and well-being. As the CEO of your health, you need to create sustainable practices that become part of your lifestyle.

Essential Long-Term Habits:

Continuous Learning: The field of health optimization is evolving rapidly. Commit to staying informed about new developments and opportunities.

Regular Monitoring: Establish routines for tracking your health metrics and adjusting your approach based on results.

Stress Management: Develop and maintain effective stress management practices that work for your lifestyle and personality.

Sleep Optimization: Prioritize sleep quality and create consistent habits that support restorative rest.

Movement and Exercise: Find forms of physical activity you enjoy and can maintain long-term.

Nutritional Awareness: Develop understanding of how different foods affect your body and energy levels.

Social Support: Cultivate relationships with people who support your health goals and understand your commitment to optimization.

CONNECTING WITH DR. JAN'S SERVICES

If you're ready to begin your optimization journey or want to explore advanced approaches like peptide therapy, I invite you to learn more about the services we offer at Viva La Skin and through our educational platforms.

Available Resources:

Comprehensive Consultations: We offer detailed assessments that examine all aspects of your health and create personalized optimization plans.

Peptide Therapy Programs: Access to high-quality peptide protocols with proper medical supervision and monitoring.

Educational Courses: For healthcare providers interested in learning about peptide therapy and optimization medicine.

Peptide Products: Through peptideadvantages.com, we provide access to pharmaceutical-grade peptides with proper quality assurance.

Ongoing Support: Continuous monitoring, adjustment, and support throughout your optimization journey.

Aesthetic Integration: Combining health optimization with aesthetic treatments for comprehensive wellness and confidence.

YOUR NEXT STEPS

Reading this book is just the beginning of your optimization journey. Here are the practical next steps to transform this knowledge into results:

Immediate Actions (Next 30 Days):

- Complete a comprehensive health assessment including advanced lab work
- Evaluate your current lifestyle habits and identify areas for improvement
- Research qualified providers in your area or consider consultation options
- Begin implementing basic optimization strategies (sleep, nutrition, stress management)

Short-Term Goals (Next 3-6 Months):

- Work with a qualified provider to develop a personalized optimization plan
- Implement initial interventions and begin monitoring progress
- Address any obvious deficiencies or imbalances identified in your assessment
- Establish sustainable habits that support your optimization goals

Long-Term Vision (Next 1-5 Years):

- Achieve your specific health and performance goals
- Develop expertise in your own health optimization
- Build a lifestyle that supports long-term vitality and well-being
- Consider advanced interventions like peptide therapy as appropriate

THE TRANSFORMATION AWAITS

Everything you need to transform your health and vitality is available right now. The science exists, the treatments are accessible, and qualified providers are ready to guide you through the process. What's required is your decision to stop accepting "normal" as optimal and start pursuing the vitality and performance you deserve.

My own transformation from obese and prediabetic to optimal health proves that remarkable change is possible at any age. But it requires taking ownership of your health, working with qualified providers, and committing to the process of becoming your best self.

You have one life to live, and your health is the foundation for everything else you want to achieve. Your relationships, your career, your adventures, your legacy—everything depends on having the energy, vitality, and mental clarity that comes from optimal health.

The question isn't whether transformation is possible—it's whether you're ready to become the CEO of your own health and commit to the journey of optimization.

Your best self is waiting. The tools and knowledge exist to help you get there. The only question remaining is: when will you begin?

To learn more about peptide therapy and health optimization, visit peptideadvantages.com or reach out to our team at Viva La Skin. Your transformation starts with a single decision—the decision to stop settling for normal and start pursuing optimal.

The future of your health is in your hands. Make it extraordinary.

CONCLUSION
MEDICINE REIMAGINED

"We stand at the threshold of a new era in human health—
one where aging gracefully isn't just hope, but science;
where feeling optimal isn't luck, but strategy; where
thriving isn't reserved for the few, but available
to anyone willing to embrace what's possible."

A S I WRITE THESE FINAL WORDS, I'M FILLED WITH EXCITEMENT about what lies ahead. Not just for you as you begin or continue your optimization journey, but for all of us as we collectively reimagine what healthcare can and should be. We're witnessing the birth of a new paradigm—one that will fundamentally change how we approach human health, aging, and potential.

The journey we've taken together through these pages mirrors the evolution happening in medicine right now. We started with the limitations of traditional, disease-focused care. We explored the revolutionary potential of peptides and integrative medicine. We examined how true health optimization requires addressing the whole person—body, mind, and spirit. And we discovered how taking ownership of your health can transform not just how you feel, but how you experience every aspect of your life.

THE PROMISE OF PRECISION MEDICINE

The future I envision isn't some distant fantasy—it's emerging right now, in practices like ours and in research laboratories around the world. We're moving rapidly toward an era of precision medicine where treatments are customized based on your unique genetics, biochemistry, lifestyle, and goals.

Imagine a world where:

- Your genetic profile guides personalized nutrition recommendations that optimize your energy, mood, and performance. Where peptide therapies are precisely calibrated to your individual needs and monitored in real-time through wearable technology. Where hormone optimization isn't guesswork but science-based precision that helps you feel your absolute best at any age.
- Where artificial intelligence analyzes thousands of biomarkers to predict and prevent health issues before they develop. Where aging isn't something that happens to you, but something you actively manage and optimize. Where the distinction between healthcare and self-care disappears because prevention and optimization become the foundation of how we maintain our most precious asset—our health.

This isn't science fiction. The foundational technologies and approaches already exist. What we're witnessing now is their integration and refinement into comprehensive systems that can help anyone achieve levels of health and vitality that previous generations could only dream of.

112

THE BIO-INDIVIDUAL REVOLUTION

One of the most exciting aspects of this new paradigm is its recognition that every person is unique. The old model of medicine assumed that everyone with similar symptoms should receive similar treatments. The new model recognizes that optimal health is deeply personal and requires individualized approaches.

Your optimal hormone levels might be different from someone else's. Your genetic variations might require specific nutrients in forms that others don't need. Your stress response patterns might benefit from peptides that wouldn't be appropriate for someone with different physiology. Your aesthetic goals and timeline might call for a completely different integration of treatments than what works for others.

This bio-individual approach means that there's no single "right" way to pursue optimization. There are principles and frameworks—like the five-pillar approach I've developed—but the specific implementation must be tailored to your unique situation, goals, and circumstances.

This is what makes working with qualified practitioners so crucial. It's not enough to follow generic protocols or copy what worked for someone else. True optimization requires the expertise of providers who understand how to assess your individual needs and create personalized strategies that evolve as you progress and as our knowledge advances.

FROM MY TRANSFORMATION TO YOURS

My personal journey from obese and prediabetic at 47 to achieving what people now call "Greek statue status" represents more than just one person's health transformation. It represents proof of concept for what's possible when we embrace this new paradigm of medicine.

When I started my optimization journey, I was skeptical about many of the approaches I now use with patients every day. I had been trained in traditional medicine, and the idea that someone could fundamentally transform their health, body composition, and vitality through integrative approaches seemed too good to be true.

But the results spoke for themselves. The comprehensive testing revealed the root causes of my symptoms. The targeted interventions—hormone optimization, genetic-based supplementation, peptide therapy, and lifestyle modifications—produced measurable improvements in every aspect of my health. The transformation wasn't just physical; it was mental, emotional, and spiritual.

More importantly, it ignited a passion for helping others achieve similar transformations. Every patient who goes from feeling terrible despite "normal" labs to experiencing optimal health validates this approach. Every person who discovers their energy, confidence, and vitality through optimization becomes proof that this new paradigm of medicine works.

If a physician who had let his health deteriorate to the point of obesity, prediabetes, and crushing fatigue could achieve such transformation, then anyone can do it with the right approach, qualified guidance, and commitment to the process.

THE RIPPLE EFFECT OF OPTIMIZATION

The impact of health optimization extends far beyond individual transformation. When you feel your best, you show up differently in every area of your life. Your relationships improve because you have more energy and emotional resilience. Your career advances because you have better focus, creativity, and stress tolerance. Your family benefits because you're more present, engaged, and capable of enjoying shared experiences.

This creates ripple effects that extend through families, communities, and society as a whole. Children who grow up seeing their parents prioritize health and vitality learn to value these things themselves. Workplaces benefit from employees who are energetic, focused, and resilient. Healthcare systems benefit when people require less treatment for preventable chronic diseases.

As more people embrace optimization and take ownership of their health, we create a cultural shift toward prevention, vitality, and personal responsibility that benefits everyone.

THE INTEGRATION OF AESTHETICS AND LONGEVITY

One of the most exciting developments in this new paradigm is the recognition that how we look and how we feel are intimately connected. The integration of aesthetic medicine with health optimization isn't vanity—it's comprehensive wellness that addresses both internal vitality and external confidence.

When you look in the mirror and see someone who appears healthy, vital, and confident, it affects every aspect of how you experience life. This is why the work we do at Viva La Skin, combining cutting-edge aesthetic treatments with comprehensive health optimization, represents the future of medicine.

True beauty isn't about conforming to artificial standards or trying to look decades younger than your chronological age. It's about looking like the healthiest, most vibrant version of yourself at any age. It's about the confidence that comes from knowing you're taking care of yourself and investing in your long-term health and vitality.

THE DEMOCRATIZATION OF ELITE HEALTH

What excites me most about this revolution is how it's making elite-level health optimization accessible to anyone who's committed to pursuing it. Tools and treatments that were once available only to professional athletes or the ultra-wealthy are now within reach of anyone who prioritizes their health.

Comprehensive genetic testing costs less than a weekend getaway. Advanced lab work that provides detailed insights into your hormone levels, inflammatory markers, and nutritional status is available at reasonable prices. Peptide therapy, hormone optimization, and other cutting-edge treatments are offered by qualified providers throughout the country.

The information and education needed to make informed decisions about your health are freely available. Wearable technology provides real-time feedback on your sleep, stress, and recovery. Online platforms connect you with experts and resources regardless of your geographic location.

This democratization means that your zip code, income level, or social connections don't have to determine your access to optimization. What matters is your commitment to pursuing it and your willingness to work with qualified providers who can guide you through the process safely and effectively.

YOUR ROLE IN THE REVOLUTION

You are not just a beneficiary of this medical revolution—you're a participant in it. Every person who chooses optimization over disease management, who takes ownership of their health rather than remaining a passive patient, who demands better from their healthcare providers and themselves, is helping to drive this transformation forward.

By purchasing this book, you've already taken the first step. By implementing the principles and strategies I've shared, you become part of the solution. By working with qualified providers who understand optimization rather than just disease treatment, you support the growth of this new paradigm.

By sharing your transformation with others—your increased energy, improved body composition, enhanced cognitive function, or renewed confidence—you inspire others to pursue their own optimization journey.

This is how revolutions happen: one person at a time, one transformation at a time, one decision at a time to stop accepting "normal" as optimal and start pursuing what's truly possible.

YOUR NEXT CHAPTER BEGINS NOW

The knowledge you've gained from this book is valuable, but knowledge without action is just entertainment. Your transformation begins the moment you decide to move from reading about optimization to actually pursuing it.

Start with the fundamentals: comprehensive assessment of your current health status, identification of your specific goals and priorities, and connection with qualified providers who can guide you through the process. Begin implementing basic optimization strategies while you develop your more comprehensive plan.

Don't try to change everything at once. Build gradually, monitor your progress, and adjust your approach based on results. Remember that optimization is a journey, not a destination, and that the most sustainable transformations happen through consistent, incremental improvements over time.

Most importantly, embrace the mindset shift from patient to CEO of your health. Take ownership of your well-being, make informed decisions about your care, and never settle for feeling suboptimal when the tools and knowledge exist to help you thrive.

RESOURCES FOR YOUR JOURNEY

To support you in this journey, I've created several resources that can help you implement the strategies and principles we've discussed:

Peptide Advantages (https://peptideadvantages.com): Our comprehensive platform for high-quality peptides, educational resources, and support for your optimization journey. Here you'll find pharmaceutical-grade compounds with proper quality assurance, detailed information about different peptides and their applications, and guidance for working safely with these powerful tools.

Viva La Skin: Our integrated aesthetic and wellness center where we combine advanced cosmetic treatments with comprehensive health optimization. This is where the future of medicine is being practiced today—addressing both internal vitality and external confidence through science-based approaches.

Educational Courses: For healthcare providers interested in learning about peptide therapy and optimization medicine, we offer comprehensive training programs that cover both the science and practical application of these approaches.

Consultation Services: Whether you're local to our Myrtle Beach location or need remote guidance, we offer consultation services that can help you develop and implement your personalized optimization strategy.

THE FUTURE IS NOW

The future of medicine isn't coming—it's here. The tools, knowledge, and qualified providers exist right now to help you achieve levels of health, vitality, and performance that would have seemed impossible just a generation ago.

Peptides represent just one category of these revolutionary tools, but they exemplify everything that's exciting about this new paradigm: precision targeting of specific biological processes, working with your body's natural systems rather than against them, customizable protocols based on individual needs, and the potential to optimize rather than just treat.

As our understanding of human biology continues to advance, as technology provides ever more sophisticated ways to monitor and optimize our health, and as more providers embrace this integrated approach to medicine, the possibilities will only expand.

But you don't have to wait for some future breakthrough. Everything you need to begin your optimization journey is available right now. The question isn't whether transformation is possible— it's whether you're ready to begin.

A PERSONAL INVITATION

This book has been my attempt to share not just information, but inspiration. To show you what's possible when we embrace a new paradigm of medicine that focuses on optimization rather than just disease management. To demonstrate through science, patient stories, and my own transformation that remarkable change is possible at any age and any starting point.

But ultimately, your transformation is up to you. You can read about optimization, or you can pursue it. You can remain a passive patient in the traditional medical system, or you can become the CEO of your own health. You can accept "normal" as optimal, or you can discover what you're truly capable of achieving.

I invite you to choose optimization. I invite you to take ownership of your health and commit to the process of becoming your best self. I invite you to join the revolution that's reimagining what's possible for human health and vitality.

Your best self is waiting. The tools and knowledge exist to help you get there. The only question remaining is: are you ready to begin?

Visit https://peptideadvantages.com to take the first step in your optimization journey. Connect with our team at Viva La Skin to explore comprehensive assessment and personalized protocols. Join the thousands of people who have already discovered what it means to truly thrive.

The future of your health starts now. Make it extraordinary.

Dr. Solomon Jan, MD
Founder, International Society of Aesthetic and Regenerative Medicine
Medical Director, Viva La Skin
https://peptideadvantages.com

APPENDICES
REFERENCES & GLOSSARY

COMPREHENSIVE PEPTIDE REFERENCE GUIDE

This reference guide provides an overview of the major peptide categories and their primary applications. Always work with a qualified medical provider before considering any peptide therapy.

GROWTH HORMONE-RELEASING HORMONES AND PEPTIDES (GHRH/GHRP)

Primary Function: Stimulate natural growth hormone production

Key Peptides:
- **Sermorelin**: Most studied GHRH, identical to first 29 amino acids of natural GHRH
- **CJC-1295**: Long-acting GHRH with extended half-life
- **Tesamorelin**: FDA-approved for HIV-associated lipodystrophy
- **Ipamorelin**: Selective GHRP with minimal side effects

- **Hexarelin**: Potent GHRP with additional cardiovascular benefits
- **Ibutamoren (MK-677)**: Oral growth hormone secretagogue

Typical Applications: Anti-aging, body composition improvement, muscle growth, fat loss, sleep enhancement, skin quality, recovery optimization

TISSUE REPAIR AND HEALING PEPTIDES

Primary Function: Accelerate healing and tissue regeneration

Key Peptides:
- **BPC-157**: "Body Protective Compound" for comprehensive tissue healing
- **TB4/TB4 Active Fragment (Ac-SDKP)**: Thymosin Beta-4 for soft tissue repair
- **Vilon**: Immune system support and tissue protection
- **Epithalon**: Telomere support and cellular longevity
- **Pinealon**: Pineal gland support and circadian rhythm optimization
- **DSIP**: Delta Sleep-Inducing Peptide for sleep and recovery
- **AOD-9604**: Growth hormone fragment targeting fat metabolism
- **GHK-Cu**: Copper peptide for wound healing and skin regeneration

Typical Applications: Injury recovery, chronic pain, gut healing, post-surgical recovery, anti-aging, skin health

COGNITIVE ENHANCEMENT AND NEUROPROTECTIVE PEPTIDES

Primary Function: Support brain health, memory, and cognitive function

Key Peptides:
- **Cerebrolysin (IV and oral/CerebroPep)**: Neuroprotective and cognitive enhancement
- **Semax**: Nootropic peptide for focus and memory
- **Selank**: Anti-anxiety and cognitive support
- **BPC-157**: Also crosses blood-brain barrier for neuroprotection
- **TB4 Active Fragment (Ac-SDKP)**: Supports neuroplasticity
- **DSIP**: Improves sleep quality and brain recovery
- **Humanin**: Mitochondrial support and neuroprotection
- **SS-31**: Mitochondrial peptide for energy and brain function

Typical Applications: Memory enhancement, focus improvement, anxiety reduction, neuroprotection, brain injury recovery, age-related cognitive decline

IMMUNE SYSTEM MODULATING PEPTIDES

Primary Function: Balance and optimize immune function

Key Peptides:
- **Thymosin Alpha 1 (TA1)**: Immune system regulation and viral defense
- **TB4 Active Fragment (AGES)**: Anti-aging and immune support
- **Zn-thymulin**: Zinc-dependent immune peptide
- **Delta Sleep Inducing Peptide (DSIP)**: Sleep and immune recovery

- **GHK-Cu**: Immune modulation and tissue repair
- **Cerebrolysin**: Immune system and brain health support

Typical Applications: Immune system optimization, viral resistance, autoimmune support, recovery enhancement, general wellness

GASTROINTESTINAL AND GUT HEALTH PEPTIDES

Primary Function: Heal digestive tract and support gut-brain axis

Key Peptides:
- **BPC-157**: Comprehensive gut healing and protection
- **TB4 Active Fragment (Ac-SDKP)**: Intestinal tissue repair
- **KPV**: Anti-inflammatory peptide for gut health
- **DSIP**: Gut-brain axis support through improved sleep
- **GHK-Cu**: Wound healing including intestinal tissues
- **LL-37**: Antimicrobial peptide for gut health
- **Tuftsin**: Immune system support in gut tissues
- **Livagen**: Liver protection and detoxification support
- **Larazotide**: Potential support for gluten sensitivity

Typical Applications: Leaky gut syndrome, inflammatory bowel conditions, digestive disorders, gut-brain axis optimization, liver health

MITOCHONDRIAL AND CELLULAR ENERGY PEPTIDES

Primary Function: Enhance cellular energy production and mitochondrial function

Key Peptides:
- **MOTSc**: Mitochondrial-derived peptide for energy and metabolism
- **SS-31**: Stabilizes mitochondrial membranes and improves function
- **Humanin**: Protects mitochondria from oxidative stress
- **5-amino-1MQ**: Supports cellular energy and metabolism
- **BPC-157**: Also supports mitochondrial function
- **TB4 Active Fragment (Ac-SDKP)**: Cellular repair and energy
- **Small-humanin-like peptides (SHLP)**: Mitochondrial protection
- **DSIP**: Cellular recovery through improved sleep
- **Melatonin**: Antioxidant and mitochondrial protection

Typical Applications: Chronic fatigue, energy optimization, exercise performance, anti-aging, metabolic disorders

SLEEP AND CIRCADIAN RHYTHM PEPTIDES

Primary Function: Optimize sleep quality and circadian rhythms

Key Peptides:
- **DSIP**: Delta Sleep-Inducing Peptide for deep sleep
- **Epithalon**: Pineal gland support and circadian optimization
- **Pinealon**: Pineal gland peptide for sleep regulation
- **Growth Hormone peptides**: Enhance natural GH release during sleep
- **Selank**: Reduces anxiety for better sleep
- **BPC-157**: Supports overall recovery including sleep
- **Melatonin**: Natural sleep hormone (technically not a peptide but often grouped)

Typical Applications: Insomnia, sleep quality improvement, jet lag, shift work adaptation, recovery optimization

AESTHETIC AND ANTI-AGING PEPTIDES

Primary Function: Support appearance, skin health, and cosmetic goals

Key Peptides:
- **GHK-Cu**: Copper peptide for skin regeneration and hair growth
- **Growth Hormone peptides**: Body composition and skin quality
- **Epithalon**: Cellular anti-aging and longevity
- **BPC-157**: Skin healing and overall tissue health
- **TB4**: Tissue repair including skin and hair
- **AOD-9604**: Targeted fat loss without growth hormone effects
- **Melanotan**: Tanning peptide (use with extreme caution)

Typical Applications: Skin health, hair growth, body composition, anti-aging, wound healing, cosmetic enhancement

WEIGHT MANAGEMENT AND METABOLIC PEPTIDES

Primary Function: Support healthy weight loss and metabolic optimization

Key Peptides:
- **GLP-1 Receptor Agonists**: Appetite regulation and blood sugar control
- **AOD-9604**: Growth hormone fragment for fat metabolism
- **Growth Hormone peptides**: Body composition improvement

- **Tesamorelin**: Specifically targets visceral fat
- **MOTSc**: Metabolic regulation and energy balance

Typical Applications: Weight loss, diabetes management, metabolic syndrome, body composition improvement

APPENDIX B
FDA REGULATORY GUIDELINES AND LEGAL CONSIDERATIONS

Understanding the regulatory landscape is crucial for safe and legal peptide use. This appendix provides essential information for patients and providers.

CURRENT FDA STATUS OF PEPTIDES

Important Disclaimer: Most peptides used for health optimization are not FDA-approved for these specific applications. This doesn't mean they're unsafe, but it does mean they exist in a complex regulatory environment that requires careful navigation.

FDA-Approved Peptides (Limited List):
- **Sermorelin**: Approved for growth hormone deficiency in children
- **Tesamorelin**: Approved for HIV-associated lipodystrophy

- **GLP-1 Receptor Agonists**: Several approved for diabetes and obesity (Ozempic, Wegovy, etc.)
- **Calcitonin**: Approved for osteoporosis
- **Insulin**: The original peptide hormone therapy

Research Peptides: The majority of peptides used in optimization medicine are available as "research chemicals" or "for research purposes only." This designation allows qualified medical providers to use them in clinical practice while staying within legal boundaries.

LEGAL FRAMEWORK FOR PEPTIDE USE

Compounding Pharmacy Regulations:

- Peptides must be obtained from FDA-regulated compounding pharmacies
- 503A compounding pharmacies can prepare patient-specific prescriptions
- 503B facilities can prepare larger batches with more stringent oversight
- All reputable pharmacies provide Certificates of Analysis (COAs) proving purity and potency

Medical Supervision Requirements:

- Peptide therapy should always be conducted under qualified medical supervision
- Physicians can prescribe compounded peptides for off-label uses based on their clinical judgment
- Patient assessment, monitoring, and safety protocols are essential

- Detailed documentation and informed consent are recommended

Interstate Commerce Considerations:

- Peptides cannot be sold as dietary supplements
- Marketing claims about treating specific diseases may trigger FDA enforcement
- "Research purposes only" labeling helps maintain regulatory compliance
- Telemedicine prescribing must follow state and federal guidelines

QUALITY ASSURANCE AND SAFETY STANDARDS

Essential Quality Markers:

- **Certificate of Analysis (COA)**: Must show purity (typically >95%), potency, and absence of contaminants
- **Proper Storage**: Peptides require specific temperature and handling conditions
- **Sterility Testing**: Injectable peptides must be tested for bacterial contamination
- **Stability Data**: Information about peptide degradation over time
- **Chain of Custody**: Documentation of handling from manufacture to patient

Red Flags to Avoid:

- Peptides sold without prescriptions
- Suppliers who cannot provide COAs

- Products marketed with specific disease treatment claims
- Extremely low prices that suggest poor quality
- Suppliers operating outside regulated pharmacy frameworks

WORKING SAFELY WITH PEPTIDES

Provider Qualifications:

- Board-certified physicians with experience in peptide therapy
- Training in hormone optimization and integrative medicine
- Established relationships with reputable compounding pharmacies
- Proper monitoring and safety protocols
- Clear communication about risks and benefits

Patient Responsibilities:

- Honest disclosure of medical history and current medications
- Compliance with monitoring requirements
- Proper storage and administration of peptides
- Prompt reporting of any side effects or concerns
- Regular follow-up appointments and lab work

Monitoring and Safety Protocols:

- Baseline comprehensive lab work before starting therapy
- Regular monitoring based on specific peptides used
- Documented assessment of benefits and side effects
- Dose adjustments based on patient response
- Clear protocols for discontinuation if needed

FUTURE REGULATORY OUTLOOK

Likely Developments:

- Increased FDA scrutiny of peptide marketing and distribution
- Potential approval of additional peptides for specific medical conditions
- Clearer guidelines for compounding pharmacy operations
- Enhanced quality standards and testing requirements
- Possible integration into mainstream medical practice

Staying Compliant:

- Work only with qualified medical providers
- Use reputable compounding pharmacies
- Maintain proper documentation
- Follow all medical supervision requirements
- Stay informed about regulatory changes

KEY QUESTIONS FOR PROVIDERS

Before working with any provider for peptide therapy, ensure they can answer these questions:

1. What is your source for peptides and can you provide COAs?
2. How do you determine appropriate dosing and monitoring schedules?
3. What safety protocols do you follow?
4. How do you stay current with regulatory requirements?
5. What happens if I experience side effects?
6. How do you document treatment and maintain compliance?

RESOURCES FOR CURRENT INFORMATION

- **FDA Website**: www.fda.gov (search for compounding pharmacy guidance)
- **Professional Organizations**: International Peptide Society, A4M (American Academy of Anti-Aging Medicine)
- **State Pharmacy Boards**: Regulate compounding pharmacies in each state
- **Medical Licensing Boards**: Oversee physician prescribing practices

APPENDIX C
REFERENCES AND BIBLIOGRAPHY

PEPTIDE RESEARCH AND CLINICAL STUDIES

1. Bodkin, N.L., et al. (1993). "Long-term dietary restriction in older-aged rhesus monkeys: effects on insulin resistance." *Journal of Gerontology*, 48(4), B142-B147.
2. Bowers, C.Y., et al. (1984). "Synthetic peptide that specifically releases growth hormone in vivo." *Science*, 226(4674), 663-665.
3. Chang, H.C., et al. (2010). "The role of stress in female reproduction: a review." *Human Reproduction Update*, 16(6), 725-744.
4. Guarente, L., & Kenyon, C. (2000). "Genetic pathways that regulate ageing in model organisms." *Nature*, 408(6809), 255-262.
5. Junnila, R.K., et al. (2013). "The GH/IGF-1 axis in ageing and longevity." *Nature Reviews Endocrinology*, 9(6), 366-376.
6. Khatib, N., et al. (2014). "BPC-157 promotes tendon healing and improves functional recovery after Achilles tendon

transection." *Knee Surgery, Sports Traumatology, Arthroscopy*, 22(5), 1124-1130.

7. Krivokuca, I., et al. (2008). "Stable gastric pentadecapeptide BPC 157 heals cysteamine-colitis and colon-colon-anastomosis and counteracts cuprizone brain injuries and motor disability." *Current Neuropharmacology*, 6(2), 122-129.

8. Lopez-Otin, C., et al. (2013). "The hallmarks of aging." *Cell*, 153(6), 1194-1217.

9. Mattison, J.A., et al. (2017). "Caloric restriction improves health and survival of rhesus monkeys." *Nature Communications*, 8, 14063.

10. Rudman, D., et al. (1990). "Effects of human growth hormone in men over 60 years old." *New England Journal of Medicine*, 323(1), 1-6.

HORMONE OPTIMIZATION RESEARCH

1. Abraham, G.E., et al. (2006). "Effects of bioidentical hormone replacement therapy on cardiovascular disease risk factors." *Alternative Medicine Review*, 11(3), 208-223.

2. Bassil, N., et al. (2009). "The benefits and risks of testosterone replacement therapy: a review." *Therapeutics and Clinical Risk Management*, 5, 427-448.

3. Baulieu, E.E., et al. (2000). "Dehydroepiandrosterone (DHEA), DHEA sulfate, and aging: contribution of the DHEAge Study to a sociobiomedical issue." *Proceedings of the National Academy of Sciences*, 97(8), 4279-4284.

4. Harman, S.M., et al. (2001). "Longitudinal effects of aging on serum total and free testosterone levels in healthy men." *Journal of Clinical Endocrinology & Metabolism*, 86(2), 724-731.

5. Hogervorst, E., et al. (2009). "Testosterone and gonadotropin

levels in men with dementia." *Neuroendocrinology Letters*, 30(6), 667-670.

ANTI-AGING AND LONGEVITY RESEARCH

1. Blackburn, E.H., et al. (2015). "Human telomere biology: A contributory and interactive factor in aging, disease risks, and protection." *Science*, 350(6265), 1193-1198.
2. Franceschi, C., et al. (2018). "Inflammaging: a new immune-metabolic viewpoint for age-related diseases." *Nature Reviews Endocrinology*, 14(10), 576-590.
3. Kirkwood, T.B. (2005). "Understanding the odd science of aging." *Cell*, 120(4), 437-447.
4. Longo, V.D., et al. (2015). "Interventions to slow aging in humans: are we ready?" *Aging Cell*, 14(4), 497-510.
5. Singh, P.P., et al. (2019). "The genetics of aging: a vertebrate perspective." *Cell*, 177(1), 200-220.

METABOLIC AND WEIGHT MANAGEMENT STUDIES

1. Astrup, A., et al. (2019). "Semaglutide and cardiovascular outcomes in patients with obesity." *New England Journal of Medicine*, 381(14), 1304-1313.
2. Batterham, R.L., et al. (2021). "Safety and efficacy of once-weekly semaglutide 2.4 mg for weight management: 68-week results from the STEP 1 trial." *The Lancet Diabetes & Endocrinology*, 9(9), 563-571.
3. Lean, M.E., et al. (2018). "Primary care-led weight management for remission of type 2 diabetes (DiRECT): an open-label, cluster-randomised trial." *The Lancet*, 391(10120), 541-551.

COGNITIVE ENHANCEMENT AND NEUROPEPTIDE RESEARCH

1. Gusev, E.I., et al. (2017). "Neuroprotective effects of cerebrolysin in patients with acute ischemic stroke: a randomized controlled trial." *Stroke*, 48(11), 2963-2969.
2. Pompilio, G., et al. (2020). "Thymosin β4 promotes cardiac repair and regeneration." *Annals of the New York Academy of Sciences*, 1479(1), 27-46.
3. Sramek, J.J., et al. (2002). "Review of the acetylcholinesterase inhibitor galantamine." *Expert Opinion on Investigational Drugs*, 11(10), 1415-1426.

REGULATORY AND SAFETY LITERATURE

1. FDA Guidance for Industry. (2013). "Compounding and the FDA: Questions and Answers." U.S. Food and Drug Administration.
2. FDA Guidance for Industry. (2016). "Pharmacy Compounding of Human Drug Products Under Section 503A of the Federal Food, Drug, and Cosmetic Act." U.S. Food and Drug Administration.
3. USP General Chapter <797>. (2019). "Pharmaceutical Compounding—Sterile Preparations." United States Pharmacopeia.

INTEGRATIVE AND FUNCTIONAL MEDICINE

1. Bland, J., et al. (2004). "Clinical nutrition: a functional approach." Institute for Functional Medicine.
2. Hyman, M. (2009). "The UltraMind Solution: Fix Your Broken Brain by Healing Your Body First." Scribner.
3. Jones, D.S., et al. (2010). "Textbook of Functional Medicine." Institute for Functional Medicine.

SLEEP AND CIRCADIAN RHYTHM RESEARCH

1. Hirshkowitz, M., et al. (2015). "National Sleep Foundation's sleep time duration recommendations: methodology and results summary." *Sleep Health*, 1(1), 40-43.
2. Mander, B.A., et al. (2017). "Sleep and human aging." *Neuron*, 94(1), 19-36.
3. Walker, M. (2017). "Why We Sleep: Unlocking the Power of Sleep and Dreams." Scribner.

NUTRITION AND NUTRIGENOMICS

1. Fenech, M. (2005). "The role of folic acid and vitamin B12 in genomic stability of human cells." *Mutation Research*, 475(1-2), 57-67.
2. Gomes, A.P., et al. (2013). "Declining NAD+ induces a pseudo-hypoxic state disrupting nuclear-mitochondrial communication during aging." *Cell*, 155(7), 1624-1638.
3. Kang, J.H., et al. (2009). "A diet high in folate, vitamin B6, and vitamin B12 is associated with reduced risk of colorectal cancer." *Gastroenterology*, 136(4), 1152-1159.

APPENDIX D
MEDICAL GLOSSARY AND KEY TERMS

A

Aesthetic Medicine: Medical specialty focused on improving cosmetic appearance through minimally invasive procedures and treatments.

Amino Acids: The building blocks of proteins; peptides are short chains of amino acids.

Anti-Aging Medicine: Medical approach focused on slowing, stopping, or reversing the aging process.

AOD-9604: A synthetic analog of the C-terminal fragment of human growth hormone that specifically targets fat metabolism.

B

Bioidentical Hormones: Hormones that are chemically identical to those naturally produced by the human body.

Biomarkers: Measurable biological indicators used to assess health status or disease risk.

BPC-157: "Body Protection Compound" - a synthetic peptide derived from a protective protein found in gastric juice.

C

Cellular Senescence: The process by which cells stop dividing and begin to deteriorate, contributing to aging.

Certificate of Analysis (COA): Laboratory documentation verifying the purity, potency, and safety of pharmaceutical compounds.

Circadian Rhythm: The body's natural 24-hour biological clock that regulates sleep-wake cycles and hormone production.

CJC-1295: A synthetic analog of growth hormone-releasing hormone with an extended half-life.

Compounding Pharmacy: Specialized pharmacy that creates customized medications based on individual prescriptions.

D

DHEA (Dehydroepiandrosterone): A hormone produced by the adrenal glands that serves as a precursor to other hormones.

DSIP (Delta Sleep-Inducing Peptide): A neuropeptide that promotes deep sleep and has various other physiological effects.

E

Endocrinology: The branch of medicine dealing with hormones and hormone-producing glands.

Epigenetics: The study of changes in gene expression that don't involve changes to the DNA sequence itself.

Epithalon: A synthetic peptide that may help regulate the aging process and support cellular health.

F

Functional Medicine: Medical approach that focuses on identifying and addressing root causes of disease rather than just treating symptoms.

G

GHK-Cu: A copper-binding peptide known for its wound healing and anti-aging properties.

GHRH (Growth Hormone-Releasing Hormone): Natural hormone that stimulates the release of growth hormone from the pituitary gland.

GHRP (Growth Hormone-Releasing Peptide): Synthetic peptides that stimulate growth hormone release.

GLP-1 (Glucagon-Like Peptide-1): Hormone involved in blood sugar regulation and appetite control.

H

Half-life: The time it takes for half of a substance to be eliminated from the body.

HRT (Hormone Replacement Therapy): Medical treatment involving the administration of hormones to supplement declining natural levels.

Hypothalamic-Pituitary Axis: The complex interaction between the hypothalamus and pituitary gland that regulates hormone production.

I

IGF-1 (Insulin-Like Growth Factor-1): A hormone similar to insulin that plays important roles in childhood growth and adult metabolism.

Inflammation: The body's immune response to injury or infection; chronic inflammation contributes to aging and disease.

Ipamorelin: A selective growth hormone-releasing peptide known for minimal side effects.

L

Longevity Medicine: Medical specialty focused on extending healthy lifespan and preventing age-related diseases.

M

Metabolism: The chemical processes that occur within the body to maintain life, including energy production and utilization.

MTHFR (Methylenetetrahydrofolate Reductase): An enzyme involved in folate metabolism; genetic variations can affect vitamin B requirements.

N

NAD+ (Nicotinamide Adenine Dinucleotide): A coenzyme essential for cellular energy production and DNA repair.

Neuroplasticity: The brain's ability to reorganize and form new neural connections throughout life.

Nootropics: Substances that may improve cognitive function, memory, creativity, or motivation.

O

Optimization Medicine: Medical approach focused on achieving peak health and performance rather than just treating disease.

Oxidative Stress: Damage caused by an imbalance between antioxidants and free radicals in the body.

P

Peptide: A short chain of amino acids linked by peptide bonds; shorter than proteins.

Pharmacokinetics: The study of how drugs are absorbed, distributed, metabolized, and eliminated by the body.

Precision Medicine: Medical approach that customizes treatment based on individual characteristics, including genetics.

R

Regenerative Medicine: Medical field focused on repairing or replacing damaged tissues and organs.

Research Peptides: Peptides available "for research purposes only" that are not FDA-approved for specific medical conditions.

S

Senescence: The process of biological aging and deterioration at the cellular level.

Sermorelin: A synthetic peptide that stimulates natural growth hormone production.

Synergy: The interaction of multiple elements to produce a combined effect greater than the sum of individual effects.

T

TB-500 (Thymosin Beta-4): A peptide that promotes healing and reduces inflammation in tissues.

Telomeres: Protective DNA-protein structures at chromosome ends that shorten with age.

Testosterone: Primary male sex hormone important for muscle mass, bone density, and overall vitality.

Thyroid Hormones: Hormones produced by the thyroid gland that regulate metabolism and energy production.

V

Visceral Fat: Fat stored around internal organs; associated with increased health risks when excessive.

ADDITIONAL ABBREVIATIONS AND ACRONYMS

- **503A/503B**: FDA designations for different types of compounding pharmacies
- **COMT**: Catechol-O-methyltransferase enzyme involved in neurotransmitter metabolism
- **CRP**: C-reactive protein, a marker of inflammation
- **FDA**: Food and Drug Administration
- **FSH**: Follicle-stimulating hormone
- **LH**: Luteinizing hormone
- **TSH**: Thyroid-stimulating hormone
- **SHBG**: Sex hormone-binding globulin
- **DHEA-S**: DHEA sulfate, the sulfated form of DHEA
- **Free T3/T4**: Active forms of thyroid hormones
- **HbA1c**: Hemoglobin A1c, a measure of average blood sugar over 2-3 months

This glossary provides basic definitions for educational purposes. Always consult with qualified healthcare providers for medical advice and treatment decisions.

FINAL RECOMMENDATIONS

The regulatory landscape for peptides is complex and evolving. The key to safe, legal peptide therapy is working with qualified medical providers who:

- Understand current regulations and compliance requirements
- Use only reputable, regulated compounding pharmacies
- Follow proper assessment, monitoring, and safety protocols
- Maintain detailed documentation and patient records
- Stay current with regulatory developments

Remember: peptides can be powerful tools for health optimization when used appropriately under qualified medical supervision. The regulatory framework, while complex, exists to protect patient safety and ensure quality standards.

For the most current information about peptide therapy and regulatory compliance, consult with qualified medical providers and visit https://peptideadvantages.com for educational resources and properly sourced compounds.

These appendices are provided for educational purposes only and do not constitute medical advice. Always consult with qualified healthcare providers before considering any peptide therapy.

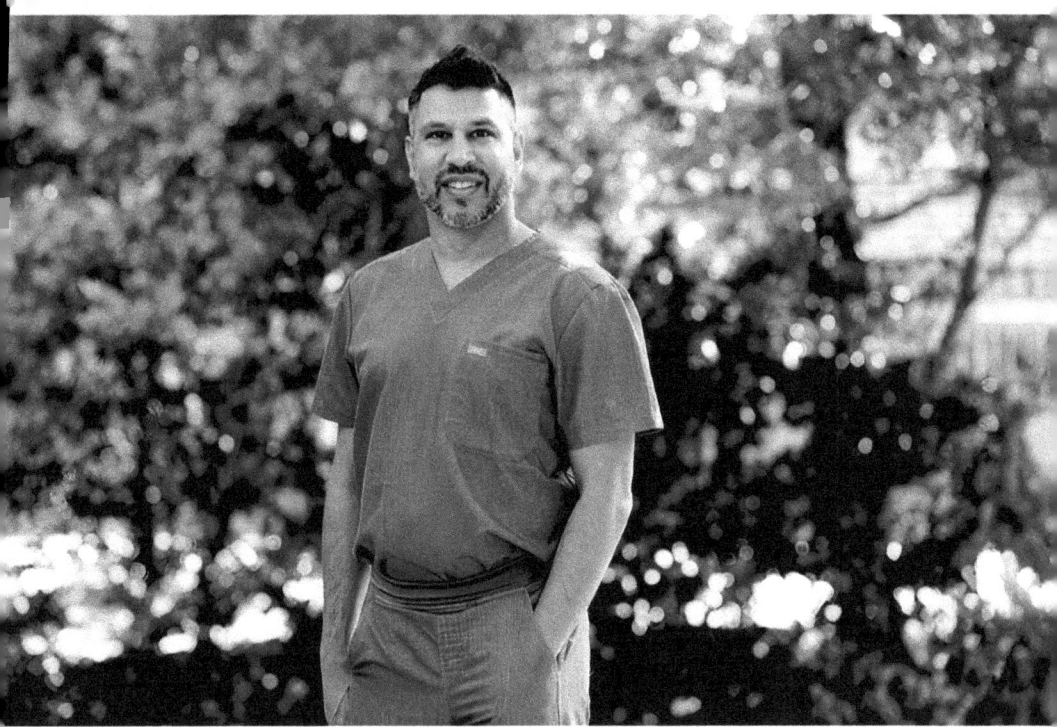

ABOUT THE AUTHOR

D R. SOLOMON JAN, MD IS A BOARD-CERTIFIED FAMILY PHYSI-
cian, Associate Professor of Medicine, and trailblazer in
integrative and regenerative care. With over two decades of clinical and academic excellence, Dr. Jan bridges conventional medicine
with cutting-edge peptide therapies to help patients and practitioners
thrive.

As Founder of the International Society of Aesthetic and
Regenerative Medicine and President of SJAN Ventures, he trains
healthcare professionals around the globe in advanced, evidence-
based protocols that deliver real-world results. Known for his
hands-on teaching style and deep clinical insight, Dr. Jan has become
a trusted mentor to a new generation of medical innovators.

From treating survivors at the Hoboken triage site during 9/11 to
serving on the front lines in South Carolina's ICUs during COVID-
19, Dr. Jan's career has been defined by courage, compassion, and an
unwavering commitment to healing.

www.ingramcontent.com/pod-product-compliance
Lightning Source LLC
Chambersburg PA
CBHW052134270326
41930CB00012B/2885